The Ultimate Parkour & Freerunning Book

Jan Witfeld, Ilona E. Gerling & Alexander Pach

THE ULTIMATE

PARKOUR & FREERUNNING BOOK

DISCOVER YOUR POSSIBILITIES

Meyer & Meyer Sport

Original Title: Parkour & Freerunning

© Aachen: Meyer & Meyer 2010

Translated by Heather Ross

British Library Cataloguing in Publication Data
A catalogue record for this book is available from the British Library

The Ultimate Parkour & Freerunning Book: Discover your Possibilities
2nd revised edition 2013
Maidenhead: Meyer & Meyer Sport (UK) Ltd., 2011
ISBN 978-1-78255-020-4

© 2011 by Meyer & Meyer Sport (UK) Ltd.
2nd revised edition 2013
Aachen, Auckland, Beirut, Budapest, Cairo, Cape Town, Dubai, Hägendorf,
Indianapolis, Maidenhead, Singapore, Sydney, Tehran, Wien
📖 Member of the World Sport Publishers' Association (WSPA)
Printed and bound by: B.O.S.S Druck und Medien GmbH, Germany
ISBN 978-1-78255-020-4
E-Mail: info@m-m-sports.com
www.m-m-sports.com

CONTENTS

Foreword 10

About this Book 14

A   THEORY 18

1   THE HISTORICAL DEVELOPMENT OF PARKOUR AND FREERUNNING 19

    1.1   Georges Hébert and His *Méthode naturelle* 19

    1.2   Educational Progressivism at the Start
            of the 20th Century and *Natural Gymnastics* 20

    1.3   Raymond Belle 22

    1.4   David Belle 22

    1.5   *L'art du déplacement* (The Art of Displacement) 23

    1.6   Naming of the Movement Art of Parkour 24

    1.7   Sébastien Foucan – From Parkour to Freerunning 24

    1.8   Definition of Parkour and Freerunning 26

    1.9   Further Development of Freerunning 26

    1.10   Outlook – Current Trends and Developments 27

    1.11   Parkour and Freerunning as Recreational, Mass and School Sports 29

2   SAFETY AND RESPONSIBILITY IN PK AND FR 31

    2.1   Belle's and Foucan's Philosophies 31

    2.2   General Behaviors in PK and FR 33

    2.3   Safety Measures and Training Rules 34

    2.4   Clothing, Shoes and More 36

3   TRAINING IN PK AND FR 39

    3.1   Basic Anatomy and Physiology 39

            3.1.1   Body Structure 39

            3.1.2   Nutrition and Energy Supply 42

            3.1.3   Physical Adaptation Processes 48

    3.2   Training Theory – Training Science 51

            3.2.1   Coordination and Technique Training 52

            3.2.2   Endurance 54

3.2.3	Strength	56
3.2.4	Speed	64
3.2.5	Flexibility	67
3.3	Training Session Organization	70
3.3.1	Warm-up	70
3.3.2	Training Emphasis	73
3.3.3	Cool Down	73
3.4	Example Exercises for Core and Supplementary Training	74

B PRACTICE 80

4	**PK & FR – BASIC MOVES**	**81**
4.1	Balancing – Équilibre	85
4.1.1	Balance Basics	86
4.1.2	Balancing on the Feet	88
4.1.3	Cat Balance (Balancing on All Fours)	89
4.1.4	Handstand (Balancing on the Hands)	90
4.2	Running – Courir	94
4.3	Jumps – des Sauts	97
4.3.1	Take-off Techniques for Support Jumps	98
4.3.2	Tic-Tac – Stepping Movements	98
4.3.3	Precision jumps – des Sauts de Précision	105
4.3.3.1 One-foot Precision		106
4.3.3.2 Two-foot Precision		108
4.3.3.3 Running Precision		110
4.3.4	Drops – Sauts de Fond	112
4.4	Landing Basics – Réception	113
4.4.1	One-footed Landings	114
4.4.1.1 Landing in the Lunge Position		114
4.4.1.2 Crane		115
4.4.2	Two-foot Landings on the Same Level and for Drops	118
4.4.2.1 Eccentric Silent Landing		118
4.4.2.2 Landing Using the Hands with Deviation to Forward Movement ("Landing and Diverting")		122
4.4.2.3 Landing and Continuing onto a Lower Level		124
4.4.2.4 Landing with Roll ("PK roll"/roulade)		126

4.5	Vaults – Passement/Passe Barrière	130
	4.5.1 Step Vault	132
	4.5.2 Speed (Vault) – Passement Rapide	134
	4.5.3 Lazy (Vault) – Passement	140
	4.5.4 Kong (Vault) "Monkey" – Saut de Chat	144
	4.5.5 Dash (Vault) – Passement Assis	152
	4.5.6 Kash (Vault)	156
	4.5.7 Reverse (Vault) – Passement Arrière	162
	4.5.8 Turn (Vault) – Demi-tour	166
	4.5.9 Palm Spin	172
4.6	Climbing – Grimper	177
	4.6.1 Wall Run/Wall-up – Passe Muraille	179
	4.6.2 Cat Leap/Arm Jump – Saut de Bras	186
	4.6.3 Muscle-up/Climb-up – Planche	192
	4.6.4 Wall Dismount	194
4.7	Hanging and swinging – Lâché	197
4.8	Underbar – Franchissement	201
	4.8.1 Feet First Underbar	201
	4.8.2 Spiral Underbar	208
5	**FREERUNNING – ADVANCED MOVES**	**213**
5.1	Loops – Culbuter	213
	5.1.1 Aerial	214
	5.1.2 Side Flip	221
5.2	Wall Tricks	226
	5.2.1 Wall Spin	226
	5.2.2 Wall Flip	234
6	**SCENE AND OUTLOOK**	**241**
6.1	Interviews with Some of the World's Best Freerunners at The Art of Motion in Sweden	241
6.2	The Scene	250
6.3	Groups	250
6.4	Workshops	251
6.5	Training and Further Education	251
6.6	Competitions	252

6.7   Clothing and Shoes 252

6.8   Miscellaneous 253

7   PARKOUR AND FREERUNNING IN SCHOOLS 255

7.1   Pedagogical Aims and Rationales for Parkour in Schools 255

7.2   Contents and Activities 259

7.3   Basic Principles of Curriculum Structure 260

7.4   Safety 264

7.5   Lesson Plans 268

       7.5.1   Basic Structures 268

       7.5.2   Six simplified example lesson plans 269

8   THE PK/FR LEXICON 281

8.1   Standing Positions Relative to the Obstacle 281

8.2   Axes of Rotation 282

8.3   Support and Hang Grips 283

       8.3.1   Support Grips 283

       8.3.2   Hang Grips 286

8.4   Glossary of Parkour and Freerunning Techniques 288

9   BIBLIOGRAPHY 304

ACKNOWLEDGEMENTS 308

APPENDIX 1 309

APPENDIX 2 310

INDEX 318

PHOTO CREDITS 327

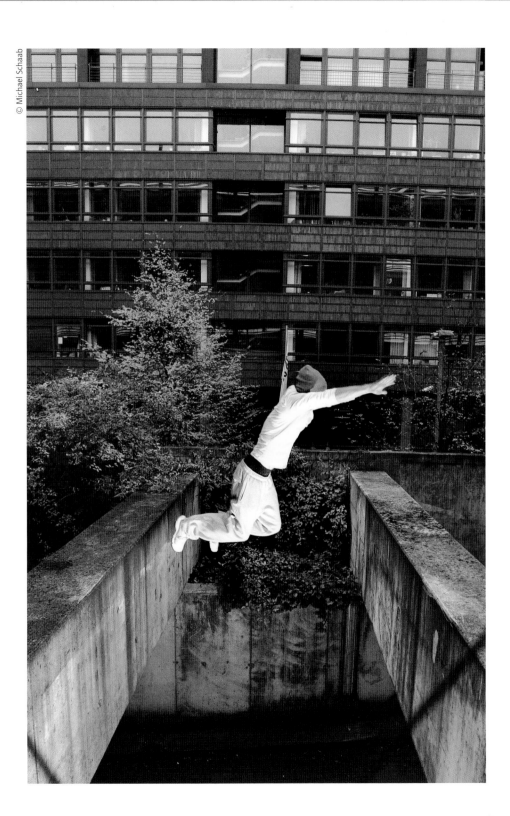

FOREWORD

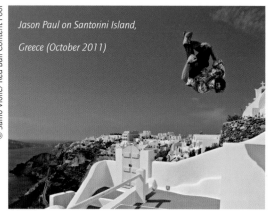

Jason Paul on Santorini Island, Greece (October 2011)

© Samo Violic/Red Bull Content Pool

We are very pleased to introduce the English language version of the book *Parkour & Freerunning – Discover Your Possibilities*. As Founders of the U.S.-based World Freerunning Parkour Federation (WFPF), we have watched with enormous satisfaction as the sport, the art and the lifestyle known as Parkour has made its way into the hearts and imaginations of Americans of all ages and backgrounds. From Sébastien Foucan's amazing opening chase scene in CASINO ROYALE to David Belle's first New York visit in 2007, to the success of the WFPF series MTV's ULTIMATE PARKOUR CHALLENGE in the summer of 2010, awareness of Parkour has been growing exponentially across America. Though we lagged behind the rest of the English-speaking world for five years or more, Americans are now making up for lost time. In fact, there are now few towns anywhere in the U.S. that can't boast at least one local freerunner testing his environment and his abilities, and posting his videos. And just try walking down the streets of New York with some of the top WFPF athletes without collecting a crowd of awestruck onlookers, as the likes of Tim Shieff, Oleg Vorslav, Jason Paul, Phil Doyle and Ben Jenkin lashay from scaffold to scaffold, flying through the air and landing in a precision on a bar ten feet off the ground! The WFPF is now a family that reaches around the world, embracing the beauty, the grace, the discipline and the philosophy of the Parkour phenomenon. We've coined a phrase that sort of sums it up for us, "Know Obstacles! Know Freedom!"

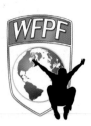

We hope this book will further your understanding of this amazing lifestyle, and the boys and girls, men and women who strive to practice it daily in all aspects of their lives.

Victor Bevine, David Thompson & Francis Lyons
Founders of World Freerunning Parkour Federation

WHAT PARKOUR MEANS TO ME

DANIEL ARROYO (USA)

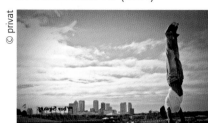

I stand with my every sense attuned to the surroundings by which I am supposed to be bound! Rapidly moving to the point that I feel the wind briefly transit across my body! My every step carefully placed so that the approach to each barrier will flow leaving no trace of fault! I run so that everything that would normally clutter the confines of my personality gives way, leaving a blissful void, the only thing in perspective the next obstacle I will overcome as I carve a path that would normally detour another! My heartbeat's rhythm is balanced with every breath and I am in rapture, distracted only by the joy of boundless freedom! In unique unison, my limbs propel me effortlessly and I know I was made to do this my whole life! In the beginning, I moved just because it was fun, but now what was once just a game has become an art that carries me through reality in a state of balanced imagination! Call it what you want, but ultimately, none of the words matter; it's the feeling that overcomes your mind that is the essence of our art of movement, this obsession that unshackles me from everything earthbound! This is the passion in which I find the love that will never let me down!

SAM KILBY (NEW ZEALAND)

Affiliate Athlete of the WFPF

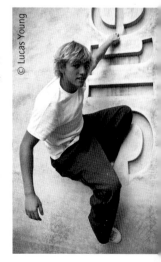

Parkour for me has been a step change in the way I view life and interact with others. It has given me discipline to train, confidence in life and myself and camaraderie with fellow participants. It allows me to be free, and express the way I feel. I learn from my mistakes allowing myself to know what I did wrong and to get back up and do it better the second time.

Parkour has given me lifelong friendships and it has allowed me to be part of a national New Zealand Team "Invictus" and also part of the WFPF (World Freerunning Parkour Federation) as an affiliate member.

Parkour is a massive part of my life and what I am most passionate about!

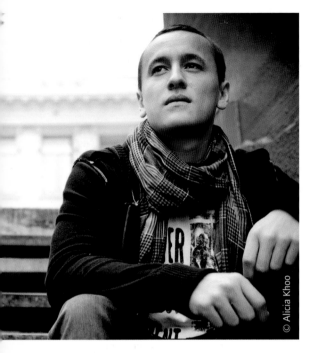

© Alicia Khoo

ETHAN SCARLETT (NEW ZEALAND)
Affiliate Athlete of the WFPF

After the passing of my sister in late 2007, I went through a lot of depression in life and was searching for something to bring me out of it. When I found Parkour, I was introduced to a new outlet for my emotions.

Parkour to me represents freedom, joy and happiness, and this is what has driven me to continue to progress through not only my environment, but also life itself. Rails, walls and rooftops are no longer boundaries, but instead have now become part of my playground. This playground also exists in my mind as I mentally push myself further than I ever thought possible. The feeling of freedom and happiness that Parkour gives me is addictive and therefore has created a new way of life for me. This way of life is agreed upon within the Parkour Community worldwide, creating a diverse and unique family bond between all practioners.

Though I may have lost one bond in my life, Parkour has helped me gain many more. To turn back now is not an option.

YOANN LEROUX (FRANCE)

For me Parkour is a life experience, an evolution which nourishes the self and the personality of the person who practices it. Above all else, it is a physical and mental method to prepare our body and spirit, which sharpens our senses of touch, sight and reflexes. The body forges and sharpens itself like a weapon which should not be used to its maximum except in the case of absolute necessity by its owner. For me, someone who uses it in all its forms, whether it be freestyle or utility, it remains for me an art, a passion, a vocation.

The generations evolve, Parkour evolves, but the basis of Parkour stays the same. At this point, we can't change the older generation, so it's up to the new generation to take up the baton and move, without any second thoughts, as a new Parkour emerges and evolves.

I can't define Parkour, or frame it, but to me Parkour means creating a mix of Urban Arts, which mix together to create one's own personal style. Martial Arts, Dance, Acrobatics all mix together with Parkour creating a kind of „sandwich" which I like to call „Free-style Parkour". Parkour is the bread and the other Urban Arts are the ingredients that you choose to put between the two slices!

And the best thing about Parkour is the „lifestyle" as we experience this lifestyle every moment, every second of the day as we are not only a family, but a community which pushes its limits whether it be against oneself or against the street.

TIM SHIEFF (UNITED KINGDOM)

Parkour to me is like flight mastery for those brief amounts of airtime that gravity allows us humans. It is total kinesthetic awareness and confidence that you have control in any situation, be it 6 inches off the ground or 15 stories up, standing, upside down or backwards. It's knowing just how long you're going to be in the air, recognizing all the different possible movements you could do with your body in that time and continuing your flow through to your landing.

Parkour in its most expressive form is the physical art created when you combine extreme environments with the limits of the human body. I've got two arms, two legs and a brain; parkour utilizes all of these, the limbs for movement and the brain for creativity. People use

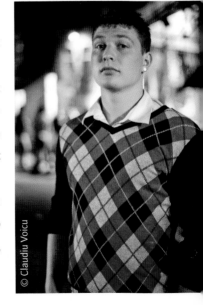

their legs to get to and from work, but in-between they forget they have them, which to me seems like such a waste when we have so much potential. Parkour is about finding that potential. I feel it has similarities with many other art forms, such as skateboarding, b-boying, capoeira. But for me the art I most like to compare it to is ballet, with its flawless fluid movement from one position to another. The main difference between the two is the speed of the movements, but when slowed down parkour can appear to be just as controlled, seamless and fluid as ballet.

Most of all, Parkour is about approaching life with a certain mental attitude, teaching you how to know your limits and how to transcend them. Parkour continues to teach me about commitment, decision-making and ironically, it keeps me grounded!

© Claudiu Voicu

ABOUT THIS BOOK

We are pleased that you have overcome the first obstacle by being interested in this book! This is a book that should help you to learn basic skills through the use of tips and photos, which can ultimately form the foundation for the discovery of the world of movement possibilities in our urban living space.

Parkour is all about the *efficient clearance of obstacles in urban and rural environments*. There are no right or wrong movements in this activity, the right solution is the one that is right for the individual.

And yet we have dared to name moves (which also have their names on the scene), to show and describe them as orientation patterns, and have also dared to reveal tips and tricks in order to teach these "models" of movement solutions for clearing man-made and natural obstacles. Starting from the origins of Parkour, methodical pointers are first given for the outdoors. Learning the basic models is essential and speeds up the learning process. Traceurs and freerunners on the scene also do this by watching videos on the Internet, (e.g., on YouTube) which feature sequences by experienced traceurs again and again, in order to copy the stars. Once you have acquired the basic movements of Parkour, you will then be free to perform experimental moves and to discover creative, unusual and individual movement solutions as situational adaptations to the features of an obstacle. By mastering Parkour-specific basic elements, you will be able to select the most appropriate move for each situation from your repertoire. Pointers on how to do this can be found in this book under the heading "Nothing is Impossible". All new moves have been named by those on the scene and can be "Googled".

Traceurs do not restrict their enjoyment of Parkour to the purely sporting aspect. Every true traceur or freerunner also lives his sport mentally and lives the philosophy of the founders D. Belle and S. Foucan, which is described from page 31 onward. This may be lost on those who only use the sporting part of the book, who are not interested in learning about and living the philosophy, which would be a shame. They should definitely try to read the theory sections of the book!

We do consider it vital though to take advantage of the excellent indoor facilities available. We are convinced that learning Parkour and especially Freerunning with the aid of apparatus, partners and safety mats will significantly increase the popularity of these "new-wave" sports.

Don't be put off by the first, thick theory section; it is best to start by looking at the fantastic photos and dipping into the movement sequences. Look for the Parkour elements that you immediately find most interesting. Read the descriptions of them and then flip through the tips and tricks and methodical suggestions. To start with, use it as a reference book for the Parkour and Freerunning elements! The longer you work with the book, the more you will also, as a Parkour or Freerunning fan, become interested in the theory, because you will want to know more and above all want to improve.

In the theory section of this book, we first want to review the origin and development of Parkour, which became known through a French youth movement and has spread throughout the world thanks to the Internet. The theory section is then devoted to training theory to help improve your performance.

But this book should, of course, first and foremost be as described above – a how-to-manual for all those who would like to try out Parkour and Freerunning. For all learners, and also for all teachers, this book offers a comprehensive methodical review of the basic techniques. Let us repeat once more: if the philosophy of Parkour and Freerunning is not the prescription of compulsory techniques, the movement solutions should therefore result in individual movement challenges with individual movement solutions, which must be

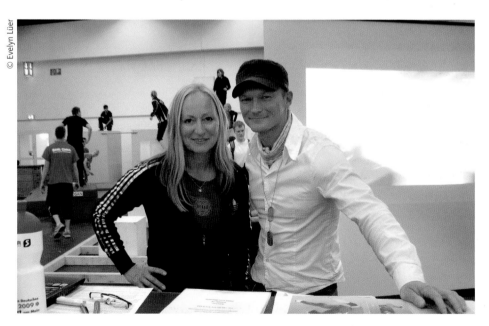

© Evelyn Lüer

Ilona E. Gerling and Alexander Pach

completely adapted to the characteristics of the obstacles. However, it is possible to provide a few methodical steps as a foundation for individual, creative performances both indoors and outdoors.

To this end, we have combined our experiences and knowledge derived from our own years of training, the exchanges within the scene, sport science education and work and from a myriad of youth and culture projects. For many years, we have been enthusiastically combining various different acrobatic styles and ways of moving and have learned a great deal during this time, of course, also from our mistakes. We have been elaborating and implementing ways of teaching Parkour and Freerunning (PK & FR) at the German Sports University Cologne since 2003 and via the platform Move Artistic at many events since 2003 too.

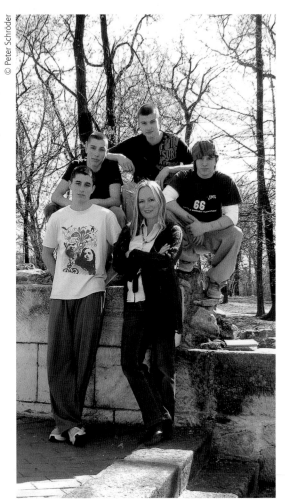

© Peter Schröder

We have now reached the point where we can properly represent the complex nature of PK & FR and its current popularity.

We do not claim that this book is complete though, for this topic and the variety of moves on the scene are too diverse. However, we would like to draw as accurate a picture as possible of this complex development process and to address the original movements and philosophies just as much as the modern forms of practicing the art of displacement.

Ilona Gerling

with Freerunners from Budapest

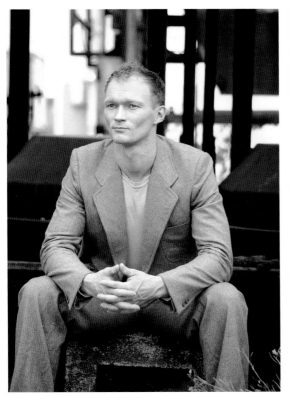

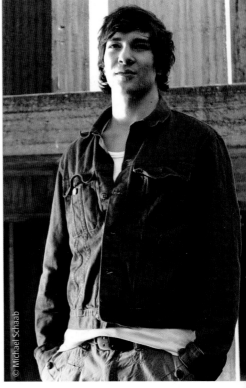

Alexander Pach

Jan Witfeld

We all have goals in our lives! In Parkour and Freerunning, the way or the movement is the goal. The obstacles represent ever-changing challenges. These challenges not only expose our personal physical limitations but also show us the possibilities and skills that can very easily be developed by motivation, concentration and repetition. To what extent this can influence people's lives is shown by many young PK and FR practitioners. This can be seen at the end of the book in the interviews with those who have dedicated their lives to Parkour and Freerunning.

Discover the unlimited possibilities within you and with Parkour and Freerunning!

Jan Witfeld   Ilona Gerling   Alexander Pach

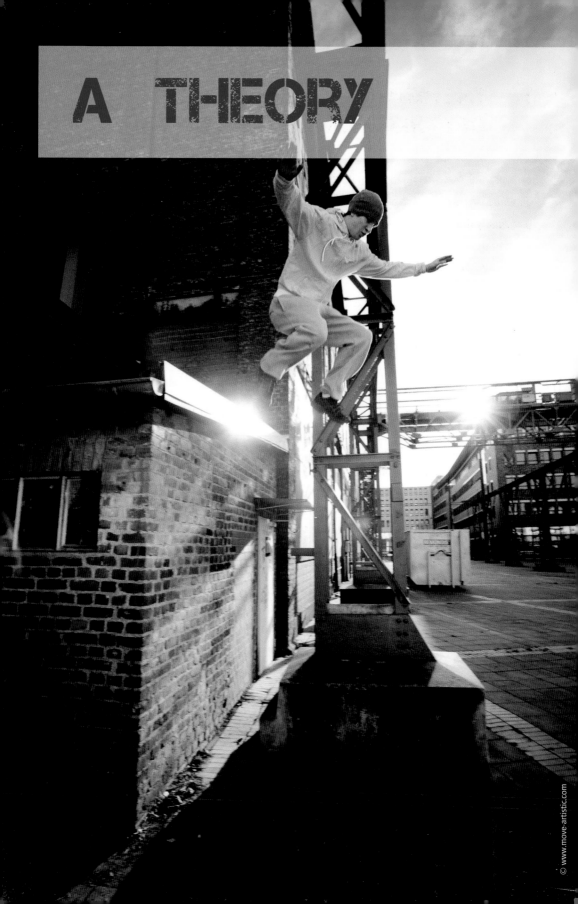

A THEORY

1 THE HISTORICAL DEVELOPMENT OF PARKOUR AND FREERUNNING

Parkour and Freerunning both originated in France. Both movement philosophies were developed in a small group of young people and spread around the whole world via the media, particularly the Internet. David Belle, a Frenchman, is credited with being the founder of the Parkour movement (Archard, 1998; Desbois, 1999). Sébastien Foucan is considered to be the founder of Freerunning.

The historical development of Parkour and Freerunning is multi-facetted and features many influential figures. We would like to start the historical development with the *méthode naturelle*, a training method that is seen as the physical and mental training foundation of the movement art of Parkour.

1.1 GEORGES HÉBERT AND HIS *MÉTHODE NATURELLE*

The historical development of Parkour begins with the training method, *méthode naturelle* (natural method), which is often seen as the philosophical foundation of Parkour also (Desbois, 1999; Foucan, 2008; Atkinson, 2009).

The *méthode naturelle*, also called *hébertisme*, sprang up at the start of the 20th century in the training philosophy of the French naval officer Georges Hébert (1875-1957). He was an advocate of life-long physical training, because he wanted people to be agile and useful in the community. Hébert was particularly impressed by the physical and mental abilities of the people from the African continent, whom he had met during his travels. "He realized that solely living in and with nature had made these people's bodies flexible, resilient and robust and their movements seem nimble and agile" (Hess & Hess, 2007 – Parkour Association Germany).

In 1902, Hébert was stationed on the island of Martinique when the region was victim of a volcanic eruption. Hébert single-handedly coordinated the evacuation of almost 700 people from a nearby village. This experience made a deep impression on him and reinforced his belief that physical strength and skill must go hand in hand with courage and altruism in order to be useful for the community (Atkinson, 2009).

After returning to France, Hébert taught at the University of Reims, where he led his then-groundbreaking, physical culture lifestyle. His training consisted of running, jumping, climbing, balancing, throwing, lifting, self-defense and swimming. However, he did not teach these physical skills separately, but taught his students in natural terrain, combined with a 5-10km endurance run.

Hébert was convinced that training the movement forms in varied, natural surroundings would enable his students to be able to use endurance, strength and speed in every geographical terrain and in any situation. He regarded competition as a distraction from the central philosophy of his training principles (Hess & Hess, 2007). In order to teach his training principles, he went on to develop a series of drills and equipment that supplemented natural conditions.

Georges Hébert was thus one of the first to popularize the training of movement techniques and physical training on an obstacle course for non-military purposes.

The modern sub-cultural term Parkour accordingly has its roots (see Fig. 1, page 25) in Hébert's use of the term "parcours" (Atkinson, 2009) and in the term of the French military *Parcours du combattant* (assault course) (Foucan, 2008). The modern image of the discipline of Parkour can therefore also be seen as a particular urban interpretation of the training principles developed by George Hébert.

In fact, the *méthode naturelle* as a training method had a strong influence on the military training of soldiers in the 1960s. During the Vietnam War, French soldiers were inspired by Hébert's training methods and his philosophy of physical, mental and emotional development. They used this principle to perfect their escape techniques in the jungle (Atkinson, 2009).

One of these soldiers was the young Raymond Belle, the father of David Belle (see Chapter 13).

1.2 EDUCATIONAL PROGRESSIVISM AT THE START OF THE 20TH CENTURY AND *NATURAL GYMNASTICS*

The educational progressivism of 1890-1940 (in which Georges Hébert was also working in France [1875-1957]), involved the reform of educational concepts affecting education both inside and outside schools. It was an international phenomenon, which began to develop specifically in industrialized countries and urban cultures. The main focus of these efforts was the child. Children should no longer be *objects* of education; instead the *individuality* of every single child should henceforth be the priority. It should be a *child-centered education*, in which the development of pupils' responsibility and autonomy were the educational goals. Its objectives should not be just the education of the mind but the development of all the children's potential.

The Games and Sports Movement in Europe was a departure from the strict, systematic gymnastics exercises in schools found around 1920 to the concept of physical education, which was intended to improve the development of children's latent movement potential, abilities and skills. Children's natural need to move was the starting point for a new kind of movement education.

The progressive educational concept of natural gymnastics and physical education developed by Austrian school reformers Karl Gaulhofer (1885-1941) and Margarete Streicher (1891-1985) quickly caught on in Germany. "The aim was no longer just to do gymnastics, to swim, run and throw with the correct style... instead the pupils should be able to develop their own abilities and skills in specific movement tasks" (Krueger, 2002, page 24).

The progressive educational principles promoted "child and nature-appropriateness" of the movement tasks, emphasized the individualization (in the context of community education) and prioritized the self-guided learning of the pupil. The real educational goal of natural gymnastics was a physical activity that educated the whole person.

Movement tasks should also stimulate creativity, and incorrect movements were even welcomed as opportunities "to discover the validity of expediency." Gaulhofer wrote, for example: "In natural jumping training, one must at all costs avoid forcing the pupil to jump in a certain way, before he has been given the opportunity for a richer movement experience" (Gaulhofer & Streicher, 1930, page 131).

In Germany, the new "physical education" was welcomed by gymnasts, because it meant a return to the old educational ideals of gymnastics of GutsMuths and Fr. L. Jahn, in which pupils did not just have to reproduce pre-determined movement patterns, as in rigid competitive and artistic gymnastics. Instead, they touted the education of the young people through movement tasks determined by the individual and corresponding to and shaping his whole personality. Natural gymnastics originated from the (natural) movement forms of running, jumping, balancing and climbing. Natural movement tasks involve every pupil creatively discovering his own individual movement solutions, which brings us back to the French contemporary Georges Héber and those who came after him, to the founders of modern Parkour: Raymond Belle and his son David (also French).

1.3   RAYMOND BELLE

Raymond Belle was born in modern Vietnam, where he was orphaned. Already as a schoolboy (at the "l'école des enfants de troupe de Dalat"), he was trained as a soldier for the French army. Around the age of 12, with some friends, he practiced and experimented with **efficient escape techniques** in order to improve his chances of survival during the war in his homeland.

These outstanding physical abilities acquired in childhood enabled him to find a job and a career with the Paris Fire Brigade as a young adult. Here he received many awards and became a role model for his two sons, Jean-François and David Belle (Belle, J-F, 2006 – Internet Blog "Parkour by David Belle").

1.4   DAVID BELLE

David Belle, son of Raymond Belle, was born on April 29, 1973 in Fécamp, France. He was raised by his maternal grandfather. The men in his family had served in the Paris Fire Brigade for generations, and he was constantly reminded of his father's extraordinary physical abilities and heroic fire-fighting deeds.

As a child, David Belle practiced gymnastics and track and field, but he always preferred to train in the open air and the woods. For him, the movements had to have an element of "usefulness" just as his father had told and explained to him. As a child, he imagined situations in which he had to put his courage and strength to the test.

His passions were overcoming obstacles, always moving forward and not letting anything get in his way. The constant running, jumping, climbing and balancing formed the foundation for his physical abilities. The physical challenges that he set himself during his imaginary stories formed the foundation for his powerful concentration.

At the age of 15, Belle relocated with his family to Lisses, near Evry, about 35 miles from Paris. There, he transferred the techniques he had learned in the forests of Normandy to the urban environment and architecture. His active, public example sparked the interest of other young people around him (Hess & Hess, 2007 – Parkour Association Germany; Belle, J-F – Homepage of David Belle: http://kyzr.free.fr.davidbelle/).

David Belle and Sébastien Foucan met at this time. What started off as playful games of chase among young people developed, during the years that followed, into a real sporting challenge: escape techniques over obstacles. The movement forms inspired by the urban landscape were further developed by this small group of youngsters, who constantly increased heights and distances, each in his way bringing something new to the movement forms. The art of displacement, or *l'art du déplacement* therefore originated from a kids' game, which was already given the name *(le) parcours* in 1989 (Foucan, 2008).

The urban, athletic movement forms first gained wide public attention thanks to a video of Belle that his brother Jean-François Belle showed to the French TV show *Stade2* in May 1997 (Belle J-F – Homepage of David Belle: http://kyrz.free.fr/davidbelle). This led to the first media reports about David Belle and his friends. In the same year, the group Yamakasi was formed by the top practitioners.

1.5   *L'ART DU DÉPLACEMENT* (THE ART OF DISPLACEMENT)

The term *l'art du déplacement* (the art of displacement) was initially used as a synonym for the word Parcours and heavily influenced by the French group Yamakasi, whose members were some of the first to develop and advance the art of displacement. The original nine members included David Belle, Yann Hnautra and Chau Belle-Dinh (Edwards, 2009, page 10).

Yamakasi's current fame and popularity in the Parkour and Freerunning scene was acquired through their mythical status as the first Parkour and Freerunning team but also through the eponymous movie *Yamakasi – The Samurai of the Modern Age* by Ariel Zeitoun and Luc Besson, which was first shown in 2001. The term *l'art du déplacement* already existed before the usual modern terms Parkour and Freerunning and is described by the English author Dan Edwardes as the original term for this movement art (Edwardes, 2009, Page 8).
Even then, Yamakasi combined efficient escape techniques with creative and acrobatic movements from other sports. The nature of the exercise and the differing approaches were reasons why David Belle and Sébastien Foucan, who was also an early member of the group Yamakasi, left the group in 1989. At this time, Belle and Foucan followed their own way to

bring about Parcours according to their individual understanding. This period is very well-documented by the French newspaper article published on October 1 by Emmanuelle Archard entitled *Les Hommes-Chats sur Bercy...* (The Cat Men of Bercy).

The group Yamakasi still exists to this day.

1.6   NAMING OF THE MOVEMENT ART OF PARKOUR

As mentioned above, Parkour was originally written in French *le parcours*. The current spelling with a "k" and without an "s" arose from a kind of separation from the existing terms *(le) parcours and l'art du déplacement*. It is speculated that David Belle coined the modern term Parkour in order to pay homage to his late father.

In this way he remembered the origins and reduced Parkour as he understood it to efficient movement and escape techniques because escape was a matter of life or death for his father as a child soldier (Müller, 2009).

In parallel to the term *l'art du déplacement*, the art of displacement, there now exists the term Parkour, which is today defined as the art of efficient movement.

At the end of the 1990s, media interest in the movement arts increased dramatically, with TV appearances and the first offers of film and advertising work. Despite this increased interest, David Belle and Sébastien Foucan went their separate ways, citing differing future plans as the reason for the split.

Belle saw his future in the movies. He learned English and took acting lessons. Foucan wanted to teach and popularize the art of displacement.

1.7   SÉBASTIEN FOUCAN – FROM PARKOUR TO FREERUNNING

In 2001, Sébastien Foucan formulated his own philosophy with the term Freerunning ("follow your way"). In some cases, this discipline was also written as Free Running. The first media references to the term Freerunning include the English documentaries Jump London (2003) and Jump Britain (2005). These documentaries, which are also considered to be important testimonials of the Parkour movement, were a milestone for the emerging Parkour and Freerunning movement in England. Inspired by the documentaries, the first English groups formed in the footsteps of Sébastien Foucan.

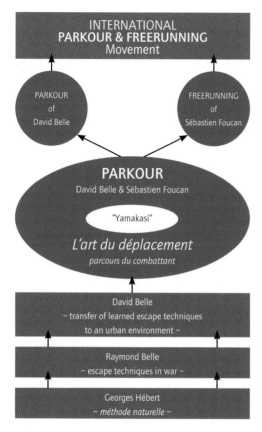

Fig. 1: Simplified representation of the developmental history of PK & FR.

There is debate over whether Foucan's term Freerunning was considered the universal term for the movement form Parkour and for *l'art du déplacement*, in order to make it more accessible to an English-speaking public, or whether Foucan even then was aiming for a separate development of the movement form of Freerunning. This is where opinions in Germany and England differ. Regardless, Sébastien Foucan is considered to be the founder of the movement discipline of Freerunning. However, author Dan Edwardes attributes the idea for the term "Freerunning" not to Foucan but to Guillaume Pelletier, who had collaborated with Foucan on the Channel 4 documentary Jump London. Furthermore, the existence of the term dates from 2003).

At this time, terminological chaos reigned. The relatively young movement forms had now spread beyond the borders of France and a varied and colorful scene had sprung up, which along with efficient escape techniques also practiced creative and acrobatic movements in urban terrain. The definition of Parkour as efficient movement by David Belle excluded acrobatic movements. Sébastien Foucan's *Philosophy of Freerunning* on the other hand offered a much more open interpretation with regard to which movements belonged to Freerunning and which did not.

This led to creative and acrobatic movements in urban settings being termed *Freerunning*.

Whether or not it was Foucan's goal right from the start to differentiate between Parkour and Freerunning is open to question. The movements that Foucan and Belle presented for their different movement philosophies are not actually that different from each other and make their common origins very clear.

Since then, Freerunning has been considered a separate discipline.

1.8   DEFINITION OF PARKOUR AND FREERUNNING

DEFINITION OF PARKOUR

Parkour is described as a movement discipline or art, in which the practitioner, called the traceur (a person who draws a line, or a path), adopts other ways than those set out for him architecturally or culturally. The traceur chooses his own way through the natural or urban space and runs along a path he sets for himself, clearing any obstacles that may arise as quickly and efficiently as possible, focusing on a controlled execution of the movements and the flow of the movement combinations. Parkour is understood to be the art of efficient movement.

DEFINITION OF FREERUNNING

Freerunning is understood as a derivative of the movement discipline Parkour. The basic movement techniques in urban and natural settings often form the foundation of Freerunning techniques and technique combinations. The emphasis though lies not on moving forward but on moving one's own body and interacting with the environment creatively and individually.

1.9   FURTHER DEVELOPMENT OF FREERUNNING

Freerunning has seen a dramatic increase in the variety of movements and movement techniques in only a short time. This can be explained by the influence from other sports.

Elements of acrobatic movements from extreme martial arts, gymnastics, Capoeira, breakdance, and tricking (tricking is a young sport movement that freely and creatively combines elements of extreme martial arts, gymnastics and other disciplines) are incorporated into the urban obstacle courses.

The free and creative nature of Freerunning has led to completely new movement creations and combinations. The diversity of acrobatic Freerunning wall tricks in particular appears now to have increased significantly.

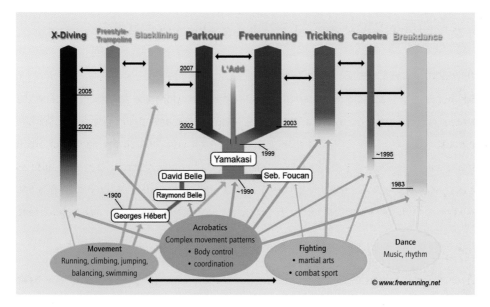

Fig. 2: Overview, origin, structure and relationship of modern movement arts (according to Müller, 2009, www.freerunning.net).

1.10 OUTLOOK – CURRENT TRENDS AND DEVELOPMENTS

Parkour and Freerunning spread from France through Europe, to the USA and Russia to the whole world. This development was massively influenced by countless media reports and scenes in world-famous movies, such as *Banlieue 13* (USA title: *District B13*) or the James Bond film *Casino Royale*, in which Sébastien Foucan appears as a freerunner in the opening scene.

Another milestone for the worldwide appreciation of the movement forms was the use of Parkour and Freerunning scenes by Madonna in two of her music videos ("Hung up" and "Jump").

Rapid global diffusion and development were aided by Internet video portals like YouTube, which provided a platform for the presentation of Parkour and Freerunning videos and enabled a rapid international exchange of experiences. Meanwhile, in other countries, numerous groups of young people were springing up, with the aim of following in the footsteps of their French heroes.

Where there is demand, there will be supply. Due to the increasing demand for clarification and training guidance, the first teams and agents at local and national levels were formed, offering training facilities and workshops. Growing international interest led to the first events and competitions.

Although neither David Belle nor Sébastien Foucan had intended Parkour and Freerunning to be competitive sports, there are now a few competitions for these target groups. The first competition of this type was the Parcouring World Championships on July 9-10, 2007 in Munich, Germany.

The competition consisted of a timed obstacle course that was promoted with Parkour images. At that time, the competition sparked a lively debate over whether Parkour competitions were going in the right direction. From this difference of opinions at that time, an interest group sprang up, which objected to Parkour in connection with competitions ("Pro Parkour, against competition").

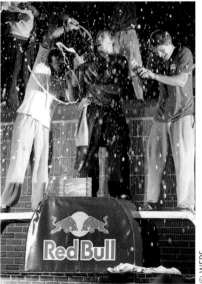

© WFPF

Although Sébastien Foucan also said that he was against competitive Freerunning, it is also developing in a different direction. On October 6, 2007, Red Bull organized the first Freerunning/Freestyle Moves Contest, called "Art of Motion," in Vienna, to which an international selection of freerunners was invited in order to establish the best freerunners by means of a one-minute "show run."

The Parcouring World Championships were likewise expanded to include a style contest for the Freerunning community in 2008. A third international competition was organized by Urban Free Flow in London in September 2008, called the Barclaycard World Freerun Championships. All three competitions were also held in 2009.

Since 2009, there has been the completion of an open air Parkour and Freerunning Park in Copenhagen, Denmark, and the first indoor training hall for Parkour and Freerunning in Russia (St. Petersburg) and in Germany (Cologne – Move Artistic Dome). Others are currently under construction. The scene is developing rapidly and diversely, and it is exciting to see which direction it will take.

1.11 PARKOUR AND FREERUNNING AS RECREATIONAL, MASS AND SCHOOL SPORTS

The disciplines of Parkour and Freerunning both have potential not only as recreational and mass sports for young people but also, and above all, as school sports. The open tasks that can be solved with basic movement forms like running, jumping, supporting, climbing, etc., combined with the limitless variety of movement combinations and the creative character of these "movement skills" all make Parkour and Freerunning desirable supplements to established school sports like track and field and Olympic gymnastics.

Furthermore, basic climbing techniques, speed, strength and balancing drills can be integrated into school sports with the motivating image of this movement art. Also, the fact that Parkour and Freerunning are not considered to be competitive sports can create a new incentive in sports lessons.

As well as school sports, there is another associated possibility of Parkour and Freerunning in youth projects and experiential education. In Parkour, it is important to be able to rely on one's own physical and mental strengths and to take responsibility for one's own actions. Physical potential and limitations can therefore be experienced directly. Quick learning success guarantees an individual sense of achievement.

One aspect that Parkour cannot teach satisfactorily is that of trust and responsibility, as in Parkour it is not usually necessary to rely on other people. This aspect is more easily found in Freerunning, where mutual aid and safety are necessary due to the complex acrobatic movements involved and also to speed up the learning process.

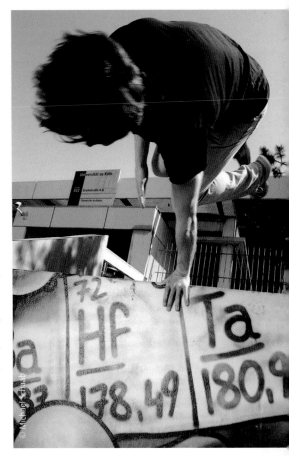

© Michael Grabb

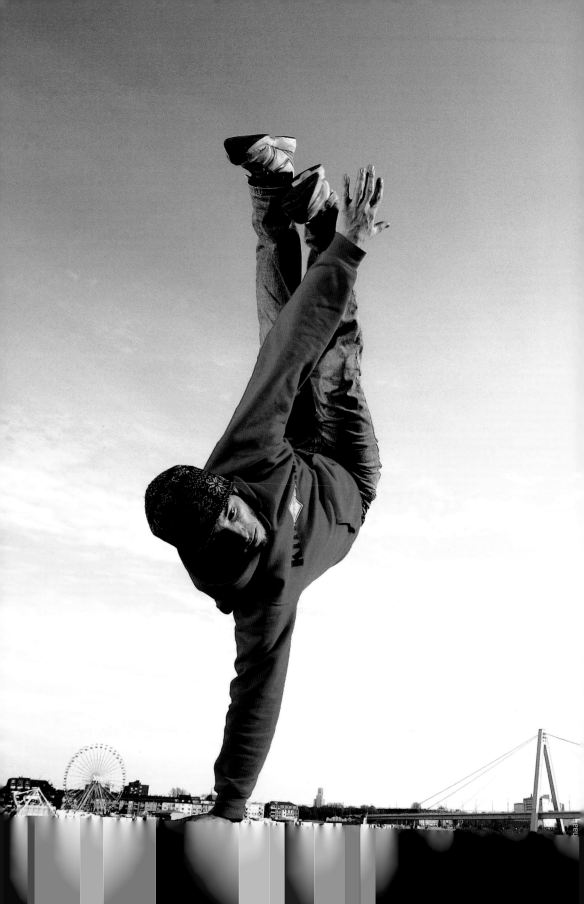

2   SAFETY AND RESPONSIBILITY IN PK AND FR

Parkour and Freerunning (hereafter referred to as PK and FR) are linked to self-confidence and physical and mental independence. Practicing them requires great responsibility, self-control and persistence. Along with the apparently unlimited movement possibilities that these movement arts offer, in return they demand a responsible attitude toward one's own health, one's fellow men and the environment.

2.1   BELLE'S AND FOUCAN'S PHILOSOPHIES

While the common origin of PK and FR is unquestioned (see Fig. 1, page 25), the movement philosophies that David Belle formulated for PK and Sébastien Foucan for FR are essentially different although they have some similarities.

For Belle, PK is a harmonious and, above all, useful way of moving in natural and urban spaces using one's own abilities. Speed, strength, endurance, body control, self-confidence and the ability to adapt to different circumstances are promoted and developed by PK. As well as striving to form one's body as a useful tool, willpower, perseverance and modesty also belong to the virtues that Belle highlights as desirable.

These virtues can also be transferred into everyday life and help to overcome the obstacles we face there. While practicing PK, Belle advises constant vigilance, for it would be catastrophic to end up disabled as an invalid in the search for absolute freedom in movement.

Foucan, on the other hand, was very strongly influenced by Asian ideologies. He created his own way from his PK roots by developing a philosophy that unifies body, spirit and environment. He called this philosophy "follow your way" or Freerunning.

His learning style is based on self-reliance, play and positive energy. Foucan presents his philosophies, thoughts and values as "Freerunning Values" on his homepage with the following messages:

Freerunning Values

Follow your way.

Always practice.

Respect others in their practice.

Be an inspiration for others.

Be positive and look for positive environments.

Respect your environment.

Feel free to try other disciplines.

Don't take it too seriously.

The journey is more inportant than the goal.

There is no good or bad, right or wrong but what is important is what you learn from your experiences through your practice.

Freerunning is not an elite discipline, but for people who love and continue to move.

Channel your energy in a good way, a way to be better.

Source: www.foucan.com (2008)

Belle and Foucan reject competition in their disciplines and encourage cooperation, which can be much more enriching.

These philosophical guidelines by the founders do not lay down laws that must be strictly adhered to. They are instead positive basic attitudes and experiences that can serve as models and should provoke reflection and discussion.

2.2   GENERAL BEHAVIOR IN PK AND FR

PK and FR are often presented on the Internet at a very high level by professional traceurs, freerunners and stuntmen. Although they are often performed with the necessary safety procedures, this is not always obvious in the clips. In addition, the pros have years of experience.

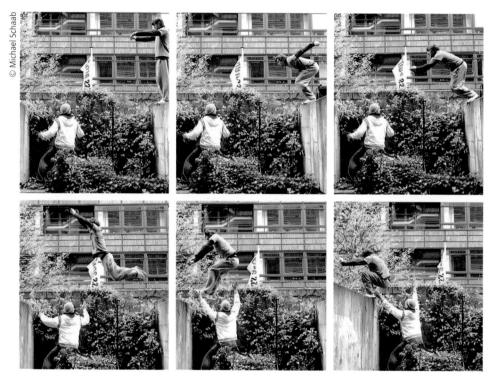

© Michael Schaab

First attempts with partner support – Gap Jump

If PK or FR are attempted alone, without experience or previous training, one should be clear that these two disciplines are very dangerous and risky and can be injurious to one's health. In addition, public or private property can be damaged by inappropriate use. However, more critical is that accidents can lead to irreversible damage through injuries and, in extreme cases of naïve, unprepared and conceited behavior, can have fatal consequences.

Based on the ideas formulated by Dan Edwardes, Susanne Pape-Kramer, the guidelines of *Parkour* by David Belle and the philosophy of Sébastien Foucan for Freerunning, the authors of this book have compiled a few important guidelines for proper behavior.

GENERAL BEHAVIOR

- *Don't take unnecessary risks: knowing one's own limits is the most important training principle. Never be swayed by peer pressure.*
- *Mutual respect: everyone can practice what he likes.*
- *Mutual support: experienced practitioners support beginners.*
- *Environment and property: the environment should not be altered or damaged. Respect private and public property.*
- *Health: treat your body mindfully and gently. Each one must take responsibility for his own health and safety. Respect your body and protect your health.*

2.3   SAFETY MEASURES AND TRAINING RULES

As well as behavior, there are a few basic safety measures that should be particularly observed by beginners.

GENERAL SAFETY AND TRAINING RULES:

- *Don't try to do too much too soon! It takes a while for your body to adapt to the physical challenges of PK and FR. Your muscles adapt relatively quickly, but don't forget that your tendons, ligaments and bones adapt much more slowly than your muscles.*
- *Create prerequisites! The human body is not very well suited to jumping onto hard surfaces, so one must first train regularly and gradually increase the load.*
- *Train close to the ground! The majority of training takes place close to the ground, where you can train all basic elements without placing yourself unnecessarily in danger.*
- *Look for support when taking your first steps! Don't train alone as a beginner; it's important that someone is present in case of an emergency. Take your cell phone with you so that you can call an ambulance if necessary.*
- *Is a first-aid kit readily available? Always have basic first-aid equipment handy (bandages, tape, cold spray, antiseptic spray).*

Further safety measures are dealt with separately in this book in the outdoor training and indoor training sections.

OUTDOOR TRAINING

In the choice of new training spots, it is important to first thoroughly investigate the terrain:

The different surfaces should be checked for unevenness and especially for broken glass. Next, the obstacles one wants to use should be checked thoroughly with the hands. Shaky ground, crumbly wall edges, sharp and rusty metal edges and unstable roofs can represent a real danger in the practicing of PK and FR techniques.

Once you have checked out the terrain and the obstacles, you can start warm-up training.

Rain and snow are other great dangers for outdoor PK and FR. Although some traceurs and freerunners train in rain or snow, see these as additional challenges and as means and technique for training your concentration and control under tougher conditions, everyone should be clear that wet surfaces represent a greater risk. The wetness will be carried around everywhere by the soles of your shoes.

Stone surfaces are often not particularly slippery, unless they are covered with moss or foliage. Metal, though, is an incalculable risk, not only in terrain, for balancing exercises and precision jumps, but also metal edges on flat roofs in wall runs or arm jumps. So, take care with wet surfaces or, even better, train under cover when it's raining!

INDOOR TRAINING

Prior indoor training can be very helpful for Parkour, especially at the school level. For the learning of complex freerunning techniques, it is almost essential. Unlike the learning of Parkour techniques, which mostly require good self-evaluation, not to mention the fact one can often feel one's way gradually into new movements, freerunning training is associated with spotting and securing. Somersaults, flips and similar tricks must first be learned through repetition.

For the practitioner, learning means not only taking a certain element of risk but is connected with certain dangers. Great responsibility is therefore required from the helper when supporting and safeguarding. The authors therefore recommend always working together with experienced freerunners/spotters when learning tricks and flips.

TIP

If there is no experienced helper present and you are learning acrobatic moves by yourself, first get an accurate view of the moves (in this book or on the Internet) and then practice the moves by jumping into water or "foam pit." These two training methods do not remove the risk of injury altogether, they just greatly reduce it.

2.4 CLOTHING, SHOES AND MORE

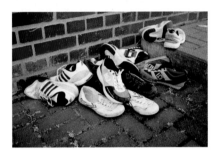

Examples of popular brands.

In order to practice PK and FR, one really only needs a pair of sneakers and general training apparel.

Most traceurs and freerunners wear conventional training apparel with shorts or long sweatpants and t-shirts, long-sleeved tees or sweatshirts/hoodies. The main thing is to be comfortable with sufficient freedom of movement. The clothing should be adapted to the weather conditions and be durable.

A beanie hat helps in cold weather so that your body doesn't lose heat too quickly. Long johns and long-sleeved tees give a little protection against grazes, e.g., when performing rolls. They also prevent dirt from getting into grazes and cuts.

As protection for the hands, cycling gloves have proven useful, especially for beginners, to avoid hurting the hands from overly rough walls, small stones on the ground or sharp edges. Cycling gloves have the advantage of leaving the fingers free thus allowing the fingers sufficient feel in order to be able to grip (e.g., to have greater control) when climbing or performing a cat leap. Wide sweatbands worn on the wrists can protect the inside of the wrists from grazes during cat leaps and wall runs.

Unlike clothing, it is a little harder to recommend shoes, as opinions are divided on this subject. Some people prefer shoes with good shock absorption for the optimal cushioning of countless landings on usually hard surfaces. Others favor a very thin sole to allow the feet more feeling. This enables better control during balancing exercises on poles and when performing precision jumps, and furthermore the foot muscles get a better workout in these more flexible shoes. Whichever shoes you choose they should have a good grip. Continuous soles have proven to be the best choice especially for precision jumps.

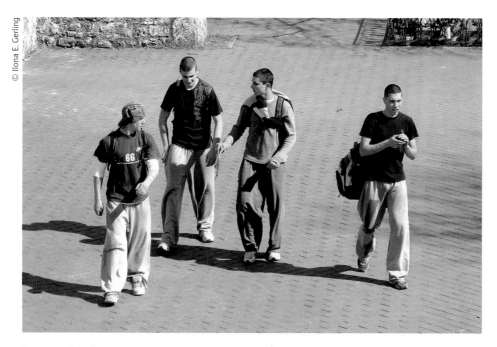

© Ilona E. Gerling

Freerunners in Budapest

We don't advise you to buy the most expensive shoes as they quickly wear out. Specially designed PK and FR shoes are usually more stable than running shoes and have better grip. In our experience, these special shoes are not necessary though to have fun practicing PK and FR.

Many traceurs and freerunners set off in the open air with a backpack containing a drink, cell phone, towel or a change of clothing and ideally a first aid kit.

For novice kids, a few authors recommend protectors. We think that it is up to parents to decide, as they know their children best. Experienced traceurs and freerunners correctly complain that protection restricts their freedom of movement. Parkour should not be seen as a crazy stunt sport, but this approach requires a certain maturity (good protection for kids/ beginners is provided by shin pads and cycling gloves, possibly also knee and elbow pads).

I (Jan Witfeld) personally must admit that after many an accident I've wished that I'd been wearing cycling gloves and shin pads.

JAN'S TIP

Heel pad shoe inserts have proven to be very useful in countless drops.

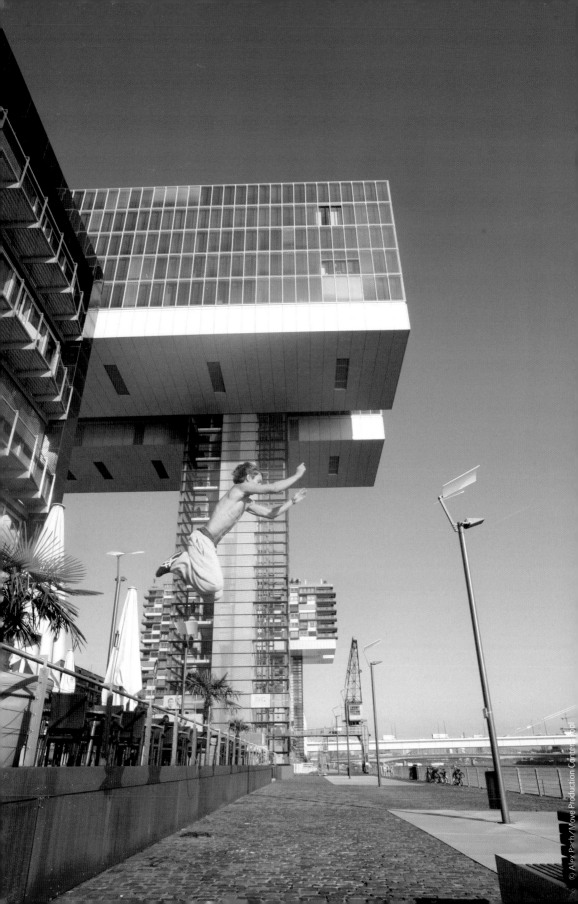

3   TRAINING IN PK AND FR

Parkour and Freerunning engage the whole body. Complex PK and FR training works all large muscle groups. But how do you train correctly? This question is not so simple, and the answer is different for everyone.

To get nearer to the answer, it is first necessary to understand a few things about the structure of the human body (anatomy) and how it works (physiology), along with energy supply and basic human adaptation processes to loading (e.g., physical activity).

3.1   BASIC ANATOMY AND PHYSIOLOGY

In this chapter, we shall take a look at the topics of anatomy (body structure) and physiology (body function) in order to give readers basic knowledge with regard to sporting performance and training load. This knowledge will lead to quicker results. If this is also simplified and limited to essentials, the basic knowledge below can also be helpful for coaches and physical education teachers in schools.

3.1.1   BODY STRUCTURE

Our body consists of a bony skeletal system that essentially determines the shape of the body and has the task of protecting the internal organs and enabling movement. Bones, joints and ligaments belong to the elements of the skeletal system and are known as the passive locomotor system. Movements are made possible by muscles, which are able to contract. The muscles are the elements of the active locomotor system. Muscles are connected to bones by tendons.

There are different types of muscles. Sporting activity primarily uses the skeletal musculature, which has the following tasks outlined below.

TASKS OF THE SKELETAL MUSCULATURE
1.   Protection and postural functions
2.   Movements in the joints
3.   Storage organs for energy reserves
4.   Keeping the body warm
5.   Angle gauge (measuring in which posture the body finds itself)

STRUCTURE OF SKELETAL MUSCLE

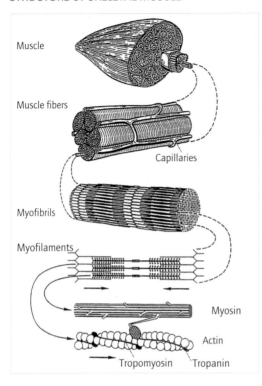

- A muscle consists of separate muscle fibers.
- Inside the muscle fibers are myofibrils, which look horizontally striped under a microscope.
- This is where the contractions take place, when actin and myosin filaments slide against each other. Energy is required for this process.

Fig. 3: Structure of a skeletal muscle (according to Markworth, 1986, page 29. In: Blum & Friedman, 1994, page 55)

A muscle can only contract (shorten) or release tension and relax. A different muscle must perform the counter movement The active muscle, whether flexor or extensor, is called the agonist The muscle responsible for the counter movement is called the antagonist. Only the coordinated interaction of the agonists and antagonists enables finely tuned and flowing movements. This interaction between agonists and antagonists is termed intermuscular coordination and is trainable by repeatedly practicing and perfecting movement sequences. This process of automatization ensures that the action of the antagonistic muscles is as unrestricting as possible.

Contractions are triggered by nerve impulses, whereby a motor nerve cell innervates (activates) several muscle fibers. The muscle fibers innervated by a motor nerve cell are called motor units. Motor nervous system protectors prevent all motor units of a muscle from being activated at the same time to avoid the overloading of muscles and tendons.

The coordination between different motor units of the same muscle is called **intramuscular** coordination. It can be improved by special training that increases power by innervating a greater number of muscle fibers simultaneously.

The coordination interaction of muscles (agonists and antagonists) and muscle groups enables movements (e.g. standing up and sitting down) or fulfils postural functions (e.g. standing). Movements and postural functions are described and characterized by the way the muscles work.

FUNCTIONING OF SKELETAL MUSCLES

Dynamic

- Overcoming (concentric), e.g., the pulling up action in chin-ups.
- Yielding (eccentric), e.g., landings.
- Yielding-overcoming (reactive), e.g., sprinting, running, take-off movements.

Static

- Maintaining posture (static), e.g., handstand

PROPERTIES OF THE SKELETAL MUSCLES

- The muscle possesses basic tension (muscle tone).
- Strength training increases the tension.
- Stretching training decreases the tension.
- There are different muscle fiber types of the skeletal muscles: slow and fast twitch.

Table 1: Simplified presentation of different fiber types of the skeletal muscles and their properties

Muscle fiber type	Slow – "red" skeletal muscle fibers "slow-twitch fibers" (type I)	Fast – "white" skeletal muscle fibers "fast-twitch fibers" (type II)
Fatigue	Able to resist fatigue (high aerobic capacity)	Quick to fatigue (high anaerobic capacity)
Aptitude	Suited to endurance performances and support/motor functions	Suited to explosive movements: jumps, landings, sprints

Several sub-groups, particularly type II fibers, have since been described (the terminology can differ according to the literature – for the terminology used here, refer to Pette, 1999. In De Marées, 2003, page 177):

Slow "red" fibers (type I)	Fast "white" fibers (type II)
	1. Type IIA fibers
	2. Type IIC fibers
	3. Type IIX fibers

Skeletal muscles always contain all fiber types. The ratio of fiber types (fast and slow twitch) varies from person to person. To start with, this individual ratio is genetically determined, i.e. some people are born with a greater proportion of fast-twitch muscle fibers than others. Secondly, this ratio can be selectively influenced by training stimuli. Trained sprinters have a greater surface area proportion of fast-twitch muscle fibers (type II) compared to trained long distance runners, who have a greater proportion of slow-twitch muscle fibers (type I).

The many fast, powerful approaches, jumps and landings in Parkour and Freerunning predominantly solicit the fast-twitch type II muscle fibers. It is great if one already has a muscular predisposition for this, but specific training can increase the volume of fast-twitch muscles. Everyone is able to improve their speed-strength by working on it.

Muscles need energy in order to contract, but how does this energy reach our muscles?

3.1.2   NUTRITION AND ENERGY SUPPLY

Muscles need energy, and our body receives this energy from vegetable and animal food. However, many people do not know how to eat correctly. Let us start with a few basic nutritional rules.

Research has shown that our so-called "civilized food" (according to De Marées, 2003, page 406):

- Is too fatty
- Contains too much animal protein
- Has too much sugar
- Has too much alcohol

In comparison, the German Society for Nutrition recommends the following 10 guidelines for a healthy diet (De Marées, 2003, page 407):

10 NUTRITIONAL RULES

- *Have a varied diet but don't eat too much.*
- *Eat less fat/fatty foods.*
- *Eat spicy but not too salty.*
- *Less sugar.*
- *More wholegrain products.*
- *Abundant vegetables, potatoes and fruit.*
- *Less animal protein.*
- *Drink sensibly.*
- *Eat smaller meals more frequently.*
- *Make your dressings tasty but use sparingly.*

People who practice sports regularly need more energy than those who are less active. It is therefore useful for athletes to know where the body and, in particular, the muscles get their energy from.

As well as vitamins, minerals and water, food contains three main nutrients that can be further processed by the body:

- Carbohydrates
- Fats
- Proteins

Carbohydrates and fats serve mainly as energy providers. The majority of the energy needed for sporting performances however is obtained from the breaking down of carbohydrates. Proteins are mainly used as cell building blocks.

The following table shows a selection of foods containing a high amount of certain nutrients.

Main nutrient	Function of the main nutrient	Selected food with *high* content of the nutrient
Carbohydrates	Energy provider	Fruits (fructose), potatoes, pasta, rice, (wholegrain) bread, granola bars
Fats	Energy provider	Vegetable oil (sunflower, olive)
Protein	Cell building block	Pork Fish Soya Milk Beans and corn (together!)

DRINKING TIP

The body heats up during exercise and starts to sweat, at which point it not only uses up energy but it also loses fluids and minerals. During training we therefore recommend a drink that contains water, minerals and fruit sugar. A suitable option is a mixture of mineral water (still or carbonated, with sodium) and a 100% fruit juice (e.g., apple juice) in the proportion of 60% mineral water and 40% apple juice.

Energy drinks are not recommended for regular consumption during training from a nutritional point of view because they contain more sugar than the body can directly consume.

HOW DO THE MUSCLES OBTAIN THE NECESSARY ENERGY FROM FOOD?

Starting in the mouth, then in the stomach and intestine, food is increasingly broken down and enters the blood stream mainly through the intestinal wall. The blood distributes the substances around the body. The substances necessary for muscle contraction also reach the muscle cells via the bloodstream.

Which substances are used in which ways by our muscle cells as energy is a science in itself. Here we try to present the processes as simply as possible.

WHICH SUBSTANCES CAN MUSCLE CELLS USE TO OBTAIN ENERGY?

The only substance that the muscles can use as an energy source is **ATP** (adenosine triphosphate).

WHERE DO MUSCLE CELLS GET ATP FROM?

The body can store a small amount of the ATP in the muscle cells themselves. Under maximal loading, this energy supply is used up within 1-2 seconds though.

ATP must therefore be continuously provided by chemical reactions (re-synthesis). The body has three different reserves for this:

- ATP/CP
- Glycogen
- Fat

In these reserves, the body has stored substances that can be converted by chemical reactions into ATP. The conversion of these substances into ATP (re-synthesis) happens in three different pathways (chemical reactions):

- Anaerobic-alactic re-synthesis = without oxygen, without lactate formation
- Anaerobic lactic re-synthesis = without oxygen, with lactate formation
- Aerobic re-synthesis = with oxygen

WHY ARE THESE RESERVES AND PATHWAYS IMPORTANT FOR US AS ATHLETES?

As described above, ATP can immediately be obtained from the first reserve (ATP/CP reserve) and by creatine phosphate (CP) be quickly replaced. This chemical reaction functions immediately, without oxygen and without lactate formation. The ATP/CP reserve is used up after 4-6 seconds under maximal loading.

The second reserve (glycogen reserve) can be used in two ways. Firstly, ATP can be obtained via a chemical reaction without oxygen. In this way, a lot of ATP can be made available in a short time. The disadvantage is that this energy supply is very wasteful. The glycogen reserve is quickly emptied and, in addition, lactate is formed as a byproduct of the chemical reaction, which with increasing blood lactate levels leads to a inhibition of the energy supply. The muscle is exhausted after 15 seconds to 2 minutes under intensive loading. You may be familiar with this state after a 440 yard sprint. It is hard to move your legs properly in the final meters, they hurt and feel very heavy.

The ATP can also be obtained from the glycogen reserves with the aid of oxygen. This allows a greater yield from the reserve because another chemical reaction takes place with the aid of oxygen. However, this reaction takes longer and cannot be used under intensive loading. The advantage is that there is no lactic acid build-up and the muscle does not get tired as quickly, thus enabling long-lasting loads of up to 120 minutes.

The third reserve (fat reserve) is almost inexhaustible. In order to form ATP though, even more oxygen is required, which must be supplied by the breathing. This form of energy supply takes a long time to kick in. This energy supply pathway only dominates in a load duration of more than 120 minutes.

The diagram below shows an overview of the energy reserves and energy production pathways.

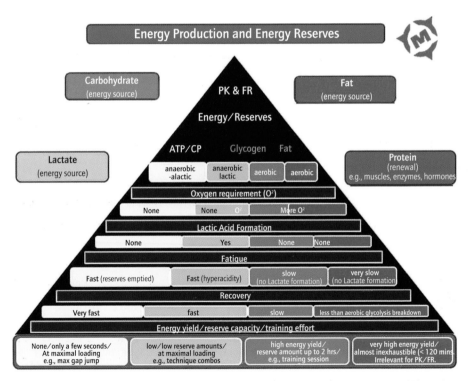

Fig. 4: Overview of the energy reserves and energy production pathways (www.move-artistic.com, adapted from Blum & Friedmann, 1994, page 29).

In reality, the energy reserves cannot be so clearly separated from each other as represented in the table. The transitions are fluid and separate from each other. That means that before one energy reserve is empty, the next-fastest energy metabolism pathway is already active.

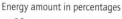
Energy amount in percentages

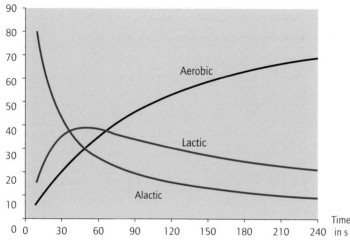

Fig. 5: Percentage amounts of alactic, lactic and aerobic energy metabolism in loading to exhaustion between 10 seconds and 4 minutes (computer simulation) (according to Heck in De Marées, 2003, page 370).

In Parkour and Freerunning, the anaerobic-alactic metabolic component guarantees the deployment of energy-rich phosphates (ATP and CP) for brief, highly intensive speed-strength efforts of a few seconds (e.g., jumps, fast accelerations). The anaerobic-lactic energy production from the glycogen reserves supports the speed-strength efforts lasting from 15 seconds to 2 minutes. Aerobic efficiency determines performance during long-lasting loads and enables a quick recovery between loads.

The ATP/CP reserves and lactate elimination require differing rest times in order to refill or break down the lactate after loading. This knowledge should be taken into consideration when structuring rest breaks in training.

If you perform short, fast/explosive loads, the necessary ATP/CP reserve is quick to refill. The half-life of the ATP/CP reserve is around 30-60 seconds (De Marées, page 363).

If you perform the same fast/explosive movements over a longer period, the anaerobic-lactic energy production from the glycogen reserve is performance-determining. Excessive lactate formation inhibits energy production and lactate elimination therefore determines the amount of recovery required. The average half-life of lactate elimination is around 15 minutes, and the speed of lactate breakdown depends on the maximal lactate value attained (De Marées, 2003, page 364).

TIP

Relaxation, combined with low-level activity, accelerates the breakdown of lactate in the blood.

3.1.3   PHYSICAL ADAPTATION PROCESSES

One characteristic of the human body is that it adapts to the demands of repeated loading (e.g., training). This can be simply illustrated by the following example: if one runs barefoot too often, the soles of the feet toughen in order to protect the feet. The skin therefore adapts to the load of barefoot running.

While lack of exercise leads to muscle atrophy, repeated loading can contribute to the maintenance or strengthening of muscles and tendons, as well as the strengthening of bones, joint cartilage and ligaments. This is most noticeable under high loads, e.g., strength training increases the muscle cross-section and thus the muscle strength. Regular strength training also gradually thickens the muscle tendons; the diameter of the long bones increases and also thickens the cartilaginous coating of the joint surfaces. Repeated stretching (not jerking!) can increase the range of movement of joints by lengthening muscles and widening cartilage-coated joint surfaces in the long term (De Marées, 2003, pages 12-13).

On the other hand, even a single excessive load can cause acute injury (e.g., strain, muscle fiber tear, break, sprain) or a chronic injury (e.g., osteoarthritis) of the musculo-skeletal system.

The resilience of physiological structures is dependent upon age, genes, gender, previous injuries, training condition; they are in a process of constant change. It is therefore in principle impossible to give a threshold value of the resilience, and it is very difficult to formulate an optimal and universally valid training program for all.

However, general training rules can be formulated as follows:

- By loading the body (e.g., training), it is possible to trigger functional adaptations. Specific loading stimuli provoke specific adaptation reactions.
- In order to trigger an adaptation, a load must exceed a certain threshold.

- Above-threshold stimuli are correct; below-threshold stimuli are ineffective, extreme above or below stimuli are damaging (Arndt-Schulzsche Rule).

Above threshold training stimuli (e.g., from strength training), initially lower the performance level. During the subsequent rest phase, the body's regeneration processes increase its performance level to a level that exceeds the starting level (supercompensation). This increased performance level corresponds in this example to an increased strength capacity.

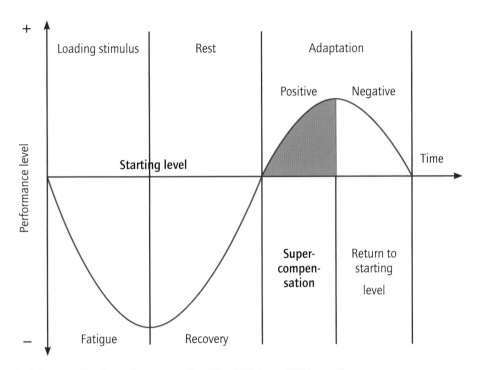

Fig. 6: Sequence of loading – adaptation reactions (Blum & Friedmann, 1994, page 6)

The pause length between consecutive training stimuli (e.g., strength training session) has a great influence on the performance level. If the rest is too short or too long, the performance level can plateau or even drop. An optimal performance increase is only possible when the new load (strength training workout) takes place at the time of highest **supercompensation** (adaptation phenomenon as higher performance capacity).

Figure 7 below illustrates this connection between loading and recovery (rest).

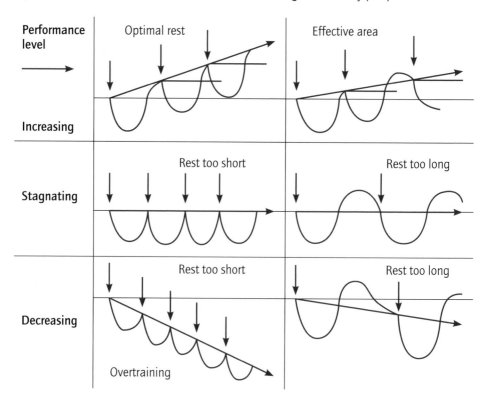

Fig. 7: Change in sporting performance level after a training load subject to rest length (after Blum & Friedmann, 1994, page 13).

The duration of the recovery process depends on the individual's fitness and the type of load.

INDIVIDUALS OF AVERAGE FITNESS CAN ADOPT THE FOLLOWING GUIDELINES FOR RECOVERY AND TRAINING EFFECT (SUPERCOMPENSATION):

- *About 72 hours recovery after strength and speed training*
- *About 36 hours recovery after endurance training.*

(Grosser et al., 1986. In Blum & Friedmann, 1994, page 6).

Various different measures (e.g., tailored nutrition, sufficient sleep, active recovery with dynamic muscle work, massage, etc.), can be employed to accelerate recovery.

3.2   TRAINING THEORY – TRAINING SCIENCE

In this chapter, we would like to outline a few basic achievements of training scientists in order to provide a concise overview and an introduction to all those who are interested as to how they can and also should train in order to achieve specific goals.

Performance in all sports is comprised of the following factors:

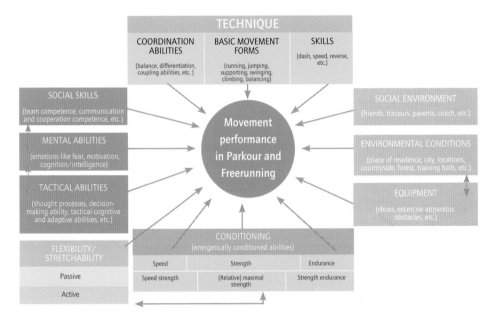

Fig. 8: *Factors influencing sporting performance in Parkour and Freerunning (modified according to Ehlenz, et al., 1985, p.12/Weineck, 2007, p.25).*

The importance of the individual components for sporting performance is different for each sport. In PK & FR, key components are those of technique as a whole, conditioning abilities (especially maximal strength, speed strength and strength endurance), flexibility and, last but not least, cognitive abilities.

How training sessions are structured in PK and FR depends totally on your personal training goals.

Training goals can include:

■   enjoying exercising and being with friends

■   learning techniques and coordination abilities

■   improving conditioning abilities (e.g., training for endurance, strength, speed, flexibility)

These personal training goals can be used to determine training content, methods and means by which the goals should be achieved.

- If the goal is to learn techniques, a sport-specific training program is required (see Chapters 4 and 5).
- If the training goal is to improve conditioning abilities, you must distinguish between the following motor core skills as they are trained differently:
  - Endurance (Chapter 3.2.2)
  - Strength (Chapter 3.2.3)
  - Speed (Chapter 3.2.4) and
  - Flexibility (Chapter 3.2.5).

3.2.1   COORDINATION AND TECHNIQUE TRAINING

Coordination skills and the mastery of sports techniques are closely linked but not the same thing.

Sports techniques are concrete actions in order to complete a movement task, while coordination skills may be called agility. They enable an athlete to master sporting movements in predictable and unpredictable situations safely and economically, in addition to learning them relatively quickly.

A broad coordination base is achieved by a variety of sports movement experiences and by the mastery of a variety of sporting techniques. For this reason, it is beneficial to try out unfamiliar sports. In children's and youth training, even for elite level youths, this should be borne in mind for a broad coordination base leads to an improved motor learning ability and aids in injury prevention (Peters, 2009, page 95; Weineck 2007, page 793 onward).

THE MOST IMPORTANT COMPONENTS

OF COORDINATION ABILITIES AND THEIR BRIEF DEFINITIONS

- **Balance ability**

  The ability to keep and regain balance
- **Orientation ability**

  The ability to adjust one's own movements to the environment and to external movements
- **Differentiation ability**

  Fine tuning and movement accuracy
- **Rhythmization ability**

The ability to understand a movement rhythm from the outside or to transfer an inner rhythm into movement

■ **Reaction ability**

Quick reactions to external signals

■ **Adaptability**

Rapid modification of planned movements in new situations

■ **Coupling ability**

Linking of partial body movements to a whole body movement

"Coordination and technique training trigger a learning process. New information is received by the brain and, once the information has been processed, causes a change in the memory structure by connecting existing structures... we call learning by interconnecting and new connections transfer learning. Transfer means that previously completed learning and exercise processes affect the result of new learning and exercise processes" (Peters, 2009, page 98 onward).

This principle of transfer learning is used for the learning and movement teaching of new techniques following methodical principles.

THE FOUR MOST IMPORTANT METHODICAL PRINCIPLES

1. From the known to the unknown

2. From the easy to the difficult

3. From the simple to the complex

4. From the slow to the fast

Movement learning may be grouped into two basic methods. Subjectively simple movements can be learned and taught simply by "showing and copying" (**holistic movement learning**). Complex movements must be separated into partial movements. These are initially taught separately and then combined into the target movement. The resulting exercise sequences are known as *methodical exercise sequences* or the **breakdown method**.

FORMS OF METHODICAL EXERCISE SEQUENCES (PETERS, 2009, PAGE 101)

■ **Principle of reducing learning aid**

The target movement is taught holistically with the aid of a support. The support is gradually reduced until the movement is successfully performed without support.

- **Principle of breakdown into functional units**

  Parts of the target movement are trained in isolation and then combined in a whole movement.

- **Principle of gradual approximation**

  Practicing of movements that are similar to the target movement in order to then be able to transfer the skills acquired to the target movement.

- **Principle of the rhythmic sequence**

  If a movement rhythm can be discerned in the target movement (e.g., in the case of take-off actions), it is then possible to carry out the target movement by working on the rhythm.

TIP

Movement learning places high demands on the nervous system, so never practice new movements when you are tired.

3.2.2   ENDURANCE

Endurance performances are characterized by the ability to produce energy over a long period of time. The intensity determines which energy metabolism is used and to what extent, which is why endurance performances are categorized by sports scientists and sports doctors according to the energy production method.

In PK and FR, people usually train in places that seem interesting for practicing the movement techniques, such as public squares with walls, railings and levels of different heights. This means that no great distances are covered, but that mainly individual techniques or short runs with movement combinations are trained. The loading duration therefore usually lies between a few seconds and, at the most, two minutes, which is followed by a rest break.

This also makes complete sense because most speed strength movement techniques in PK and FR would exhaust the necessary energy reserves at maximal intensity after short loading durations, which can lead to reduced coordination ability and concentration, thereby increasing the risk of accidents or injuries.

In PK and FR, there are no preset course lengths and there is no aim to compete with others to be the fastest. Endurance ability therefore plays a subordinate role in PK and FR.

Runs with movement combinations from 7 seconds to 2 minutes could be classified as speed endurance or short anaerobic endurance. If these runs include a lot of movement techniques that require a lot of strength, then strength endurance and speed strength endurance are dominant.

Although Parkour and Freerunning mainly involve speed strength movements, for beginners we recommend starting off with jogging in order to build a general basic endurance base. But even advanced athletes should train their basic endurance regularly by means of long runs.

POSITIVE EFFECTS OF ENDURANCE TRAINING ON THE BODY

1.   *Prevention of cardiovascular disease*
2.   *Stabilizing of the immune system*
3.   *Increase in mental resilience*
4.   *Delayed appearance of fatigue during training*
5.   *Accelerated recovery between short, fast runs*
6.   *Accelerated recovery once the training load is over*
7.   *Diminished risk of injury*

TRAINING OF BASIC ENDURANCE BY RUNNING/JOGGING (ENDURANCE METHOD)

Method	Extensive Endurance Run	Intensive Endurance Run	Regenerative Jogging
Heart Rate	140-160 bpm	160-180 bpm	Less than 130 bpm
Loading Duration	30-60 minutes	20-30 minutes	20-30 minutes

Suggested Training Frequency

- beginners: 2-3 x per week (extensive endurance run)
- advanced: 1 x per week (training supplement)

The heart rate is a way of regulating running speed. It is however only to be seen as a guide value as the heart rate is dependent upon age and changes with increasing endurance ability. As the endurance ability rises, the heart rate drops under loading due to the heart's increased stroke volume.

3.2.3   STRENGTH

In this chapter, we shall try to explain in simple steps what determines strength performances and how the musculature can be trained by strength training. The aim is to provide an approach as to how to plan and structure your personal strength training in order to improve your strength performance for PK and FR. We start below with basic explanations.

Muscle strength is the foundation for all physical movement. There are very different types of strength performance and strength abilities that can be differentiated by the type of strength and/or muscle work.

STRENGTH ABILITIES

- Maximal strength
- Speed strength
- Reactive strength
- Strength endurance

MAXIMAL STRENGTH

Maximal strength is the greatest possible strength that one can exert by means of voluntary muscle contraction.

SPEED STRENGTH

Speed strength describes the ability to move the body, parts of the body or objects at maximal speed.

Speed strength abilities may be further subdivided into starting strength, explosive strength and speed strength.

REACTIVE STRENGTH

Reactive strength means the ability to exert the highest possible concentric thrust from an eccentric movement (Schmidtbleicher & Gollhofer, 1985, page 271). Reactive muscle performances are also called stretch-shortening cycles. This form of muscle performance plays a key role e.g., in sprinting and all the jumps.

STRENGTH ENDURANCE

Strength endurance describes the ability to maintain strength performances over a long period of time (fatigue-resistance ability).

The strength abilities may be further sub-divided according to the type of muscle contraction (dynamic – static, see page 41). Figure 9 below illustrates the different strength abilities and their manifestations.

Before we describe how individual strength abilities may be specifically improved, we should first summarize the conditions that determine strength performance.

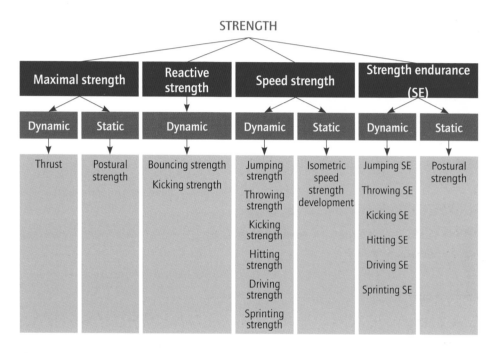

Fig. 9: Strength abilities and manifestations (according to Weineck, 2007, page 372).

Strength performance depends upon

- *Muscle cross-section (muscle thickness)*
- *Innate ratio of fast-twitch to slow-twitch muscle fibers (see page 41 onwards)*
- *Coordination of the nerve-muscle system (intramuscular coordination) (see page 40)*
- *Coordination of agonists and antagonists (intermuscular coordination) (see page 40)*
- *Type of energy supply (see page 42 onwards)*
- *Mastery of the technique corresponding to the activity*
- *Motivation and willpower*

In order to gain a thorough understanding of the effects of strength training, it is sufficient to start by understanding that strength training can trigger two main effects in the muscles:

- improved intramuscular coordination (as many motor units as possible are innervated synchronously (see page 59)
- hypertrophy (muscle build-up due to muscle fiber thickening – see below).
- Strength training initially improves intramuscular coordination, i.e., the functioning of the nerve-muscle system is optimized as more muscle fibers within a muscle are innervated simultaneously. This leads to an increase in strength. With an appropriate strength training method, an improvement in intramuscular coordination is followed by muscle fiber thickening and thus also by an increase in strength.

Figure 10 below illustrates this mechanism of strength training.

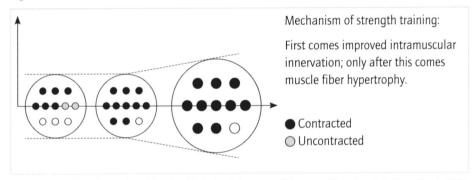

Fig. 10: Mechanism of strength training (modified after Fukanage, 1976, page 265, and quoted after Weineck, 2007, page 392).

Strength training methods that promote an increase in muscle mass are referred to as muscle building training. Muscle building is caused by training loads that exhaust the supplies of energy-rich phosphates (ATP and CP) in the muscle. In practice this means that strength exercises are performed until the musculature involved is exhausted and "no further reps" are possible.

This is, for example, achieved by dynamic strength training at moderate intensities and with many repetitions. A typical training load for beginners who want to build muscle consists of strength exercises performed slowly with 8-12 reps per set (6-4 sets) and at an intensity of 40-60% of maximal strength. Muscle building training increases muscle strength but not explosive strength in the sense of speed strength or reactive strength.

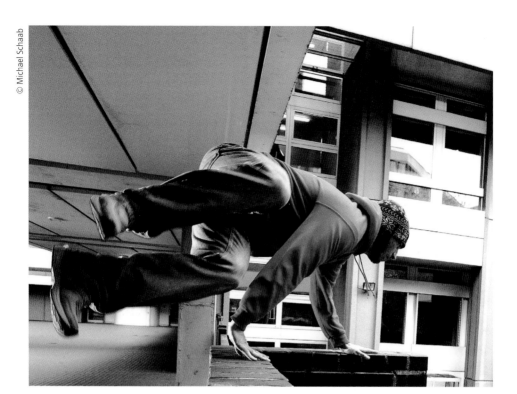

© Michael Schaab

Explosive strength is increased by dynamic or reactive strength training, i.e., performing the strength exercises at sub-maximal to maximal intensities with fewer reps in an explosive manner. These strength exercises also cause an increase in strength, but there will not be much muscle build-up. The increase in strength is achieved by an increased activation of muscle fibers and improved intramuscular coordination. This strength training method has the advantage that a greater and faster strength increase is possible without increasing bodyweight. This is useful for all athletes who want to achieve high strength performances combined with a low bodyweight (as in PK & FR). The sub-maximal to maximal intensities and the high strength peak values can however lead to muscle and tendon damage. For this reason, this high training load is not suitable for beginners. Strong muscles provide protection from injuries. Beginners, whose muscles are not well-trained, should start with a few weeks or months of muscle building training before attempting explosive strength development and a rapid increase in strength at sub-maximal to maximal intensities.

The table on the next page compares muscle building and intramuscular coordination training using dynamic strength exercises by way of example.

Table 3: Comparison of muscle building training and intramuscular coordination training during dynamic strength training exercises (modified after Blum & Friedmann, 1994, page 71).

Method (Dynamic)	General Strength training method **Muscle building training**		Special Strength training method **Intramuscular coordination training**		
Training load	Exhaustion of energy reserves (ATP & CP) by: ▪ Many reps ▪ Low intensity		▪ Few reps ▪ High to highest intensity		
Effect	Muscle fiber thickening (hypertrophy)		Synchronous employment of as many motor units as possible		
	Beginner	Advanced	Beginner	Advanced	Expert
Intensity	40-60%	60-80%	Un-suitable	80-90%	90-100%
Repetitions	12-8	10-6		6-3	3-1
Sets	6-4	8-6		8-6	10-6
Rests (between sets)	2-4 mins		3-5 mins		
Speed of movement	Slow		Fast/explosive		
Advantages	▪ Constant strength increase ▪ No high physical and mental loading		▪ High and rapid strength gain ▪ Strength gain without weight gain ▪ Explosive strength development		
Disadvantages	▪ Lower and slower strength development than intramuscular coordination training ▪ Increase in muscle tension. Stretching exercises essential! ▪ No explosive strength development possible		▪ High physical and mental loading ▪ High strength peak values under reactive loading ▪ Risk of injury! *Effective protection:* Strengthened musculature		
Use	Suitable for all sports: Beginner and advanced		Performance and elite level sports		

Now that we have described how muscular adaptations can be influenced by training load, we would like to explore in more detail the different types of strength and describe how these types of strength can be specifically improved. In the performance tips, we deliberately limit ourselves to dynamic training methods because the movements in PK & FR are predominantly dynamic, and dynamic strength performance can best be trained by dynamic strength training methods.

MAXIMAL STRENGTH

Maximal strength can be improved by muscle building training or *intramuscular coordination training*.

Method (Dynamic)	Muscle Building Training		Intramuscular Coordination training		
Performance tips for target groups	Beginner	Advanced	Beginner	Advanced	Expert
Intensity	40-60%	60-80%	Un-suitable	80-90%	90-100%
Repetitions	12-8	10-6		6-3	3-1
Sets	6-4	8-6		8-6	10-6
Rests (between sets)	2-4 mins		3-5 mins		
Movement speed	Slow		Fast/explosive		

SPEED STRENGTH

Speed strength abilities are, along with

1.   maximal strength and
2.   intramuscular coordination ability (page 40)

highly dependent upon

3.   optimal speed of movement and the interaction between the muscles engaged in the movement (intermuscular coordination) (page 40).

Speed strength abilities should therefore be trained in as discipline-specific a way as possible.

Speed strength ability and a fast-to-explosive strength development can be improved by intramuscular coordination training.

Method (Dynamic)	Intramuscular Coordination training		
Performance tips for target groups	Beginner	Advanced	Expert
Intensity		80-90%	90-100%
Repetitions	Unsuitable	6-3	3-1
Sets		8-6	10-6
Rests (between sets)	3-5 mins		
Movement speed	fast/explosive		

REACTIVE STRENGTH

Reactive (plyometric) training should, like speed strength training, always be performed in a discipline-specific manner. Reactive strength exercises also improve intramuscular coordination and the interaction between the muscles engaged in the movement (intermuscular coordination). In PK and FR, reactive strength exercises are mostly useful for improving jumping ability.

Method (Dynamic)	Intramuscular Coordination training		
Performance tips for target groups	Beginner	Advanced	Expert
Intensity	100% and over		
Repetitions	6-10		
Sets	2-3	3-5	6-10
Rests (between sets)	3-5 mins		
Movement speed	Explosive		

■ Only perform when fresh and well warmed up!

Danger of aching muscles and muscle and tendon injury

Because in our experience the question of suitable exercises for improving jumping strength is a very common one, at this point we would like to make a couple of comments about it.

Jumping strength can be improved by an increase in *speed strength* and *maximal strength*, combined with a rapid strength development and a low bodyweight. Due to the effects of coordination and movement technique on jumping performance, reactive jumping exercises have proven to be a very effective way of improving jumping strength. Figure 11 below shows examples of reactive exercises with increasing levels of difficulty to improve the reactive strength of the quadriceps muscles (at the front of the thigh) and the calf muscles when jumping.

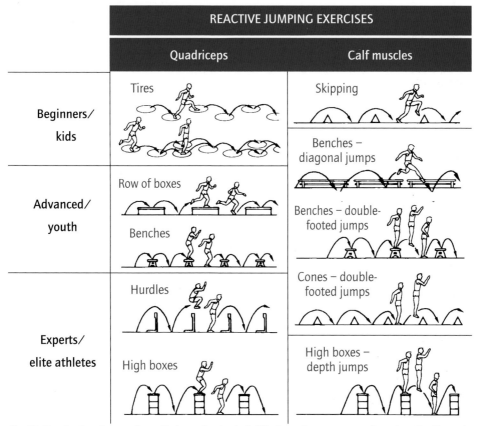

Fig. 11: Reactive jumping exercises with increasing level of difficulty to improve power of quads and calf muscles (modified after Cometti, 1988, page 136 onward, and modified after Weineck, 2007, page 448).

STRENGTH ENDURANCE

Strength endurance or speed strength endurance are trained by increasing the number of reps and the length of the training stimulus. The emphasis is on the energy supply of the desired strength, speed strength abilities, and the fast recovery of the muscles involved over a certain period of time.

However, it is difficult to formulate general performance tips for strength endurance and speed strength endurance for PK & FR because they do not take place within a specific period of time. Training for strength and speed strength endurance should be carried out in a discipline-specific manner.

In the presented training methods, we have until now limited the strength abilities to dynamic strength training methods. However, in addition to these dynamic strength training methods, there are also static (isometric) strength training methods.

Static strength training is only partly suited to PK and FR (for all dynamic sports), for static strength training has no effect on dynamic strength development, particularly not speed strength.

However, *static strength training for the core trunk muscles* is worthwhile for dynamic sports like PK and FR, because the trunk muscles have a primarily postural function. Static strength training can also be very beneficial during muscle building for the purpose of injury prevention because a small amount of this type of training can produce a rapid gain in maximal strength by hypertrophy. In addition, static training enables the muscles to be specifically solicited at desired joint angles.

CONCLUSION

PK and FR are recreational sporting phenomena, which do not involve absolute performance optimization but a movement philosophy with the aim of finding a healthy balance between body and spirit. Strength training should therefore fulfill the purpose of protecting the joints and preparing the body for loading. In addition, it can serve individual performance optimization.

3.2.4 SPEED

Speed is a complex combination of abilities that is expressed in different sports in different ways. Speed performance is, along with genetically pre-determined preconditions and conditioning abilities, highly dependent upon coordination and mental abilities. Grosser defines speed as follows:

"Speed in sport (describes) the ability, based on cognitive processes, maximal willpower and the functionality of the nerve-muscle system to achieve the highest possible reaction and movement speeds under given conditions" (after Grosser, 1991, page 13. In Weineck, 2007, page 609).

Speed can be divided into "pure" and "complex" forms (according to Schiffer, 1993. In Weineck, 2007, page 610 onward).

Pure Speed forms	Complex speed forms
Reaction speed	Speed strength
Action speed (acyclical motions, e.g., jumps)	Speed endurance (acyclical motions)
Frequency speed (cyclical motions, e.g., sprints)	Maximal speed endurance (cyclical motions)

Reaction speed describes the ability to react as fast as possible to a stimulus.

Action speed describes the ability to perform acyclical, (single motions such as jumps) at the highest possible speed.

Frequency speed describes the ability to perform cyclical, (repeated, identical motions such as sprints) at the highest possible speed.

Without going more deeply into the complex speed forms, the choice of typical examples of "pure" speed forms already shows that it is almost impossible to separate the concept of *action speed* from those of *speed strength* and *reactive strength* (see page 61 and 62), and that the boundaries between frequency speed and endurance performance ability *(speed endurance)* are blurred the longer the required cyclical speed performance must be maintained (Peters, 2009, page 131). However, there is a subtle difference, for speed performances involve not just moving fast but as fast as possible.

SPEED PERFORMANCES ARE DEPENDENT UPON:

- *A high proportion of fast-twitch muscle fibers*
- *High stimulus speed and easy nervous excitability*
- *High reserve capacity of ATP and CP in the muscle cells*
- *Good coordination, combined with mastery of the technique to be performed fast*
- *Motivation and willpower*

Speed performances are closely connected to the genetically determined fiber proportion of fast-twitch muscle fibers in the musculature. Speed is therefore a highly genetically pre-determined ability, although the period between the ages of 12 and 14 is an exception.

According to American research, at these ages, the proportion of so-called intermediate fibers (they cannot be classified as either slow or fast twitch) is relatively/proportionally high. Specific speed training can influence the transformation of intermediate fibers into fast-twitch fibers (Weineck, 2007, pages 388, 617).

As a general rule, speed can best be developed between the ages of 12 and 14. It is important to carry out a varied, age-appropriate and fun speed training with a highly challenging nature, through activities such as competitive games (tag, relay races) and team games (soccer, handball, basketball) as they are usually the most motivating.

But youths and young adults can also improve speed performance by means of intramuscular coordination training and speed drills.

PERFORMANCE TIPS FOR SPEED EXERCISES

Method (dynamic)	Repetition method Discipline-specific exercises
Intensity	Speed training is only worthwhile with maximum effort and **absolute motivation**.
Number of reps and track length	The number of reps and track length should be selected so that near the end of the exercises there is no fatigue-related drop in performance level or speed.
Rests (between sets)	Complete recovery (the recovery duration is up to the individual and dependent upon fitness; a guide is from 3-10 mins)

■ Like technique and coordination training, speed training places high demands on the nervous system, so they should only be performed when fresh and well warmed-up!

Note: It's better to complete many short workouts than a few long ones!

3.2.5   FLEXIBILITY

A wide range of motion is not only an advantage when it comes to sports movements, but it can also be important in everyday life. The range of motion is made up of the individual mobility of many joints. As children, our muscles are usually very stretchy and our joints are very flexible. With increasing age, this elasticity and joint mobility declines. "In order to maintain or increase joint mobility or to minimize the age-related loss of joint mobility, *regular stretching* is recommended" (quote from Freiwald, 2009, page 239).

The purpose of stretching exercises is primarily to maintain or improve muscle elasticity. However, when stretching the muscles, other structures are stretched also. From a sport point of view, it is not desirable to overstretch the tendons and ligaments. These structures have a stabilizing function, and destabilizing them can lead to an increased risk of injury.

From the many stretching methods, five forms of stretching exercises are described in more detail, as recommended by Freiwald (2009).

STRETCHING METHODS
- Static Stretching
- Dynamic Stretching
- Contract – Relax – Stretch
- Agonist Contract and Stretch
- Contract – Relax – Agonist Contract and Stretch

1. STATIC STRETCHING (FREIWALD, 2009, PAGE 281-283)

Execution

Careful adoption of the stretch position. The adopted stretch position is held for 5-15 seconds. Static stretches may be done alone or with a partner.

Extension

If one's aim is not just to maintain flexibility but to increase it, static stretches may be held for 15-60 seconds. The extended stretch time causes structural tissue (connective tissue) adaptations, as well as neurophysiological adaptations.

Advantages and Disadvantages

The stretch position can be controlled very easily in static stretching. When performed correctly, this stretching method is linked to discernable mental relaxation.

However, static stretching exercises appear less suited to being performed directly before maximal and speed strength movements.

2. DYNAMIC STRETCHING (FREIWALD, 2009, PAGE 281-283)

Execution

In dynamic stretching exercises, the final position is not held, but constantly extended by means of gentle bouncing. "The athlete performs 5-15 bouncing movements towards the stretch limit." The bouncing movements should be performed slowly, while increasing stretch intensity in a controlled and rhythmic manner.

Advantages

The dynamic stretching method is particularly suited to sports containing dynamic and speed strength movements.

According to Freiwald (2009, 281-83), dynamic stretching exercises (contrary to previous claims) do not trigger reflexes that could prevent optimal stretching. Healthy athletes should not suffer injuries from performing dynamic stretching.

3. CONTRACT – RELAX – STRETCH (FREIWALD, 2009, PAGE 283 ONWARDS)

In this method, the muscles to be stretched are first contracted.

Execution

The athlete starts by isometrically contracting the muscles to be stretched. The contraction should be sub-maximal to maximal and last between 2 and 10 seconds. The muscles are then relaxed and the stretch position adopted. The muscles are now stretched statically.

Advantages

The preceding contraction gives rise to great blood flow and strengthening in the musculature to be stretched. A further advantage is the increased attention that is directed to the musculature to be strengthened and stretched, which contributes to better body awareness.

4. AGONIST CONTRACT AND STRETCH (FREIWALD, 2009, PAGE 284 ONWARDS)

Execution

In this stretching method, the athlete actively assumes the final position and holds this stretch position by means of his own muscle contraction for a few seconds (less than 10 seconds). This means that the stretch position is adopted and held by the contracted agonistic musculature in order to stretch the antagonistic musculature.

Advantages

This stretching method is particularly suited to enhancing active flexibility Furthermore, the increased blood flow to and strengthening of the agonistic musculature before training and competition can be beneficial.

5. CONTRACT – RELAX – AGONIST CONTRACTAND STRETCH
   (FREIWALD, 2009, PAGE 285 ONWARDS)

Execution

The athlete first strongly (isometrically) contracts the musculature to be stretched for 2-10 seconds, then briefly relaxes the musculature and actively assumes the stretch position. By contracting the agonistic musculature, the antagonistic musculature is stretched.

Advantages

This stretching method is also an extremely effective way of developing flexibility. The increased blood flow to and strengthening of the agonistic musculature can be particularly beneficial before training and competition.

IMPORTANT TIPS (FREIWALD, 2009)

- *Always warm up before stretching.*
- *Pain must be regarded and respected as a natural limit of flexibility.*
- *Stretching to increase flexibility should (as much as possible) not be performed in the morning but in the afternoon or evening.*
- *The influence of stretching on the prevention of injuries is overestimated. Warming up and coordination training are better means of injury prevention.*
- *For immediate physical regeneration, stretching is not advisable. Loose jogging has proved to be better. Static stretching exercises can contribute to mental relaxation though.*
- *Stretching can neither prevent nor alleviate muscle soreness. Intensive stretching will even make existing muscle soreness worse.*

3.3   TRAINING SESSION ORGANIZATION

The subchapters below contain examples of how training sessions should be organized, structured and divided up. We recommend dividing into:

- **Warm-up**
    - general warm-up (jogging, games)
    - general stretching, flexibility and tension-building exercises
    - specific warm-up – preparing and attuning for sports-specific movements
- **Training emphasis**
    - this is determined by the training goals and can be implemented by various training contents, methods and means.
- **Cool-down**
    - jogging
    - static stretching exercises for solicited muscle groups ("stretching out")

3.3.1   WARM-UP

The whole body should be well warmed-up and prepared at the start of every training session. In the warm-up, one can differentiate between general activities and special sports-specific activities.

Start with a general warm-up with loose running, small games or skipping, followed by a few stretching, flexibility and tension-building exercises. These should be followed by the special warm-up with sports-specific movements.

Horst de Marées writes (see De Marées, 2003, page 565 onward) that the physiological effects of the warm-up include:

- Warming up the muscles and raising the body temperature.

- With increasing body temperature, metabolic processes in the muscles (including energy supply processes) are sped up.
- With increasing body temperature, the speed at which nerve impulses travel is sped up.
- With increasing body temperature, not only does the activity of the muscle spindles increase, but also that of the motor system in the brain, thus improving coordination, attention and reaction ability while also reducing the risk of injury.

- The increased muscle temperature also increases the contraction speed, i.e., maximal strength increases.
- The layer of cartilage thickens on the joint surfaces, thus distributing the acting forces over a greater surface area and lowering the risk of joint cartilage damage.
- Reduced likelihood of muscle, tendon and ligament tears.

The **duration and intensity** of the warm-up can only be roughly generalized. This depends on fitness, age, time of day and weather conditions.

Taking all these factors into account, the warm-up can last between 10 and 45 minutes.

GENERAL WARM-UP IN PARKOUR AND FREERUNNING

A general Parkour and Freerunning warm-up could look like this:

- Loose jogging forward, mobilizing the shoulders.
- Sidesteps with changes of direction with the arms swinging loosely by your sides.
- Leg-crossing with changes of direction, twisting the hips, with the arms and shoulders moving in the opposite direction.
- Running backwards.
- Skipping with the arms swinging loosely.
- "Heel-to-butt" kicks with running strides in-between and hip extension.
- High knees skipping to the right and left with running strides in between.
- Crouch jumps one after the other from standing.
- Short, quick accelerations.

TIP

Do not start with jumping activities or speed strength exercises (e.g., skipping)! The movement intensity should increase gradually during the warm-up.

After the general warm-up, follow with a few stretching, flexibility and tension-building exercises (see following section).

STRETCHING AND FLEXIBILITY BEFORE PK & FR TRAINING

The general warm-up is followed by a few stretching exercises.

Prior to sports that demand speed strength and maximal strength performance from the athlete, such as Parkour and Freerunning, all the musculature to be solicited in training should be pre-stretched. To this end, we recommend the following two stretching methods:

- Dynamic stretching (5-15 bouncing movements) (page 68) and
- Agonistic contract and stretch (page 69).

We advise against the static stretching method prior to training. If for personal reasons you still want to perform static stretches, make sure the stretch duration is short (less than 5 seconds in the final position).

Reason: Long static stretching before speed strength and maximal strength loading leads to a drop in performance.

SPECIAL WARM-UP

The special warm-up is connected to the general warm-up. A special, sports-specific warm-up once again specifically prepares the muscle groups to be solicited during the training session to follow. For PK & FR, a specific warm-up could look like this:

- Balancing exercises on one leg (also with the eyes closed).
- Balancing on railings.
- "Animal walk": moving on all fours (forward, backwards, sideways).
- Cat balance (see page 89 onward) on railings.
- Rolling (starting position: on all fours, standing, from small jumps).
- First jumps (concentrate on a "soft" landing).

→ *Before the first jumps, **always "activate" the core muscles!***

Example exercises: "Animal walk," "cat balance" or static strength exercises to strengthen the core muscles.

- First precision jumps (near the ground), e.g., on spots, lines, beams.
- First easy supported movements (e.g., step vault, lazy vault, turn vault; see page 132 onward).

- Hanging (cat leap/arm jump position; see page 186), combined with lateral climbing exercises on wall edges.
- Swinging on poles or branches.

3.3.2 TRAINING EMPHASIS

You must choose your own training emphasis. Just remind yourself of your training goals:

- Have fun
- Learn techniques
- Improve conditioning

Then select specific training content:

- Have fun
  - Taking into consideration your body, your environment and other people
  - With easy-to-master techniques that you can already (nearly) perform and just feel like doing.
- Learn or improve techniques
  - Select a methodology of a specific technique from chapters 4 and 5.
- Improve conditioning
  - Training of endurance, strength or speed from chapters 3.2.2 to 3.2.4.

Follow your technique and strength training with a 15 to 30 minute cool-down.

3.3.3 COOL-DOWN

Finish every workout with a cool-down.

Loose jogging is a tried and tested means of physical regeneration, as is low-intensity exercise. Stretching does not provide (immediate) physical regeneration. Many athletes report that it provides psychological and coordination benefits ("relaxation" and "loosening up") (Freiwald, 2009, page 243).

For post-training mental relaxation, we recommend static stretching of the solicited muscle groups (see page 67 onward).

Execution – Static stretching

The traceur/freerunner carefully adopts the stretch position and holds the stretch for 5-15 seconds (self-stretch or partner stretch).

Tip: You should feel no pain and the muscles should not tremble!

Extension: Hold the maximal stretch position for 15-60 seconds.

To not only retain but improve muscle elasticity, you should perform a special flexibility workout with stretching exercises (after a good warm-up) or try out holistic activities like yoga.

3.4   EXAMPLE EXERCISES FOR CORE AND SUPPLEMENTARY TRAINING

This chapter offers practical example exercises for conditioning training at home, in public places, playing fields, sports halls or in natural surroundings. Depending on your previous sporting experience, it is even advisable to start with several weeks of regular conditioning training in order to lay the foundations for outdoor PK & FR training. It is generally advisable not to limit yourself to only practicing movement techniques, but to regularly include conditioning training in your workouts.

For kids and young people in particular, we recommend bodyweight strength training without additional weights, because this permits an age-appropriate and very specific preparation of Parkour and Freerunning techniques. In bodyweight strength training, it is hard to give universally valid numbers of reps and sets for beginners, advanced, kids, youth and adults, so the example exercises are presented without specific training instructions. They are instead intended to give the reader ideas as to what core and supplementary training exercises can look like.

There is no single form of strength training that suits every target group. Every sport has its own strength demand profile. **Strength must be trained according to this demand profile.**

Depending on your goals, strength training should be general or specific and performed with high or moderate intensity or explosively or slowly.

Performance tips for improving conditioning can be found in Chapters 3.2.2 through 3.2.4.

EXAMPLE EXERCISES

The example exercises have been grouped according to the movement techniques in Chapter 4 and are offered as additional exercises. The exercises in the individual categories are arranged in increasing order of difficulty and complexity.

BALANCE

- **Balance on One Leg**
  - With the free leg make circles and Figure 8s in the air
  - Move the head to the side, up and diagonally up
  - With the eyes closed
- **Rail Balance**
  - Balance forward, backward and sideways
  - Balance forward and turn around your own (longitudinal) axis
- **Cat Balance** ⌐ balance on all fours (forward)
  - First on narrow surfaces, e.g., beams, then on railings.
- **Handstand** – keep balance on the hands.

TIP

Balance training on a "slackline" (e.g,. truck tension belt strung between trees).

RUNNING

Endurance

- **Regular running**
  - On paths
  - Cross-country over fields and woodland

Speed

- **Short sprints** (16-33 yards)
  - Short sprints in the sand
- **Sprint down** downhill paths or hills (33-66 yards) to improve frequency speed (fast stride rate)
- **Sprint up** uphill paths or hills (11-33 yards)
  - Short sprints (16 yards) will improve *acceleration speed*
  - Long sprints (66 yards) will improve *speed endurance*
  - Alternative: sprint up steps or stairs

JUMPS AND LANDING STRATEGIES

■ **Squats** two-legged (squats are exercises that train the thigh and buttock muscles)

Execution:

Feet shoulder-width apart, with the arms are folded behind the back. Now bend your knees (max. 90°) and then straighten them again. The upper body bends at the hips. Look straight ahead. The feet remain on the floor throughout the exercises.

■ Calf raises two-legged (to train the calf muscles)

Execution:

Stand with the balls of the feet on a step and raise the body using the calf muscles until you are standing on the tips of your toes. After each repetition, the heels drop below the height of the step.

■ **Two-legged Jumps up steps/stairs** (important: 6-10 jumps – run back down the steps and repeat)
  ▪ Always jump two steps at a time
  ▪ Always jump as many steps as possible
■ **Two-legged Jumps**
  ▪ Onto a knee to hip-height wall with two-footed landing. Jump down and repeat
  ▪ Onto a hip-high wall, turn around and then perform a controlled, two-footed, "soft" landing
■ Two-legged **precision jumps** with near-maximal jumping distance. Turn around and repeat – take-off and landing are roughly on the same level.
■ **"Pistols"** (one-legged squats) on a step, wall or railing.

Execution:

The free leg is extended forward. The standing leg is bent at the knee and the upper body leans forward. The standing leg also has to keep balance.

TIP

Ensure correct knee-foot alignment

- **One-legged jumps up steps/stairs**

  (6-10 jumps – run back down the steps then repeat)
  - Always jump one step at a time
  - Always jump two steps at a time
- Jumping exercises in **sand**.
- **Reactive** jumping exercises (plyometrics, see pages 62 & 63)

VAULTS

Exercises to develop supporting strength in the arms, body tension and strengthening of core muscles.

- **Core musculature** training by **static strength training exercises**.
- **Abdominal muscle training** (crunches, sit-ups) on the grass.
- **Walking on all fours** ("animal walk")
  - Forward, backward and sideways
  - Four-footed walking forward downstairs
  - Four-footed walking backward upstairs
- Different variants of push-ups

TIP

Adopt and maintain body tension! (Abdominal and buttock muscles are tensed, the body is extended)

  - Arms to the side, elbows pointing outward, hands supporting underneath the elbows
  - Arms to the side of the body, elbows pointing backward, hands support underneath the shoulders
  - Clap push-ups (to improve the rapid deployment of strength)
- In the **hanging position** (from poles or branches), raise and lower both knees
  - In the hanging position (from poles or branches), raise straight legs to hip-height and lower them slowly and under control

CLIMBING – HANGING AND SWINGING

- **On a railing**
  - Lying on your back, hang under a hip-high handrail with body tension, feet lying on the floor with legs and torso forming a straight line

Movement description:

Pull the chest to the rail and then lower yourself slowly. Change grips – overhand or underhand – or raise the feet also.

- **On a Wall Edge**
  - Hang from a wall edge in the Cat Leap Position, plant your feet against the wall and climb sideways in both directions (this can also be performed on a stair-rail).
  - From the hanging position, pull up so that you are supporting yourself, then lower yourself back to the hanging position. Repeat several times (see page 186
  - Cat Leap Position).
- **On Poles/Branches**
  - Hanging and swinging
  - Pull-up and chin-up variants:

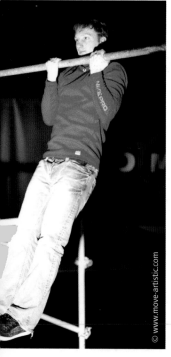

© www.move-artistic.com

  - Hands shoulder-width apart with overhand grip (thumbs pointing inward)
  - Hands next to each other with underhand grip (thumbs pointing outward)
  - Hands wide apart with overhand grip Chin above the pole Back of the neck above the pole.
  - Muscle-up (see below)

Movement description:

The muscle-up is a strength exercise for experienced practitioners. Hang from the hands (thumbs pointing in) from a pole. From the hanging position, pull yourself up (like a pull-up) and then pull yourself up into the support position (see page 192).

- **On Two Roughly Shoulder-width, Horizontal Railings or Bars**
  - Move forward, supporting yourself on your hands by moving your hands gradually forward one after the other with your legs bent.

- Supporting yourself on your hands, swing your torso and legs (rotation axes shoulders and palms of the hands, body is tensed).
- Dips (bend and straighten the arms while supporting yourself on your hands, legs bent).

■ **On a Rope**

- Climb a rope pushing up with the legs (brake and squat method). You may wear cycling gloves to protect the palms of your hands.
- For experienced athletes, use the arms only; the legs are stretched out to the sides (dangling down).

TIP

Training with a top rope anchor in the climbing gall is a very good way for both beginners and experienced practitioners to learn and perfect their climbing technique.

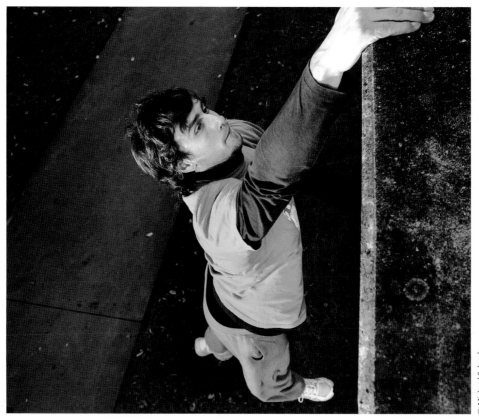

© Michael Schaab

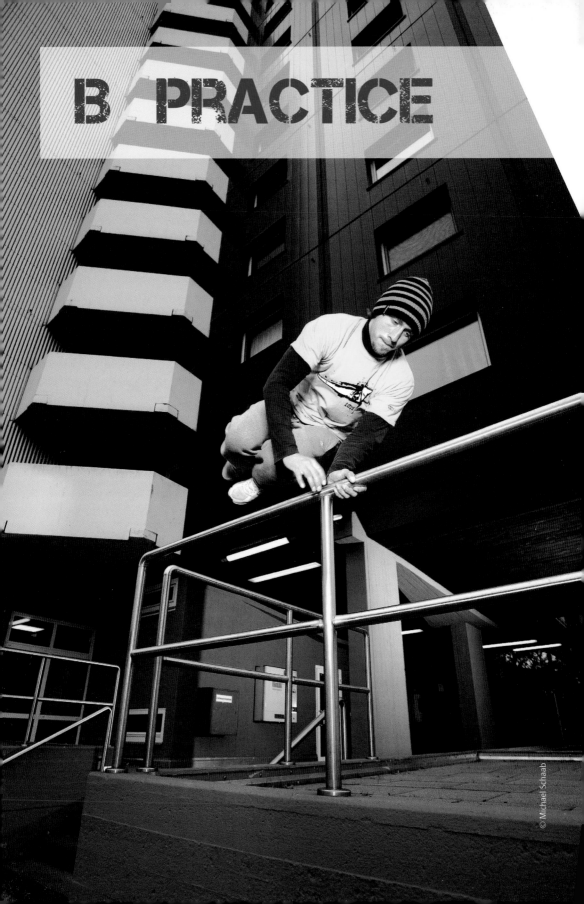

B PRACTICE

© Michael Schaab

4   PK & FR - BASIC MOVES

The basic techniques in Parkour and Freerunning are always location and object-related, or to put it more clearly, the movement techniques are dependent upon the path and obstacles selected.

Parkour and Freerunning are not disciplines with strictly predefined and standardized apparatus or obstacles nor do they have standardized techniques, instead the moves are adapted to the situation. An objective look at Parkour techniques reveals that they include man's natural movement forms, such as running, sprinting, jumping, landing, balancing, clearing, supporting, crossing, hanging, swinging and climbing.

Special variants of these basic moves can also be identified, such as a landing with a forward roll, which is a special landing technique variant of the basic landing move. A few of these techniques have already been mentioned in the movement repertoire of basic moves (such as the Kong Vault as a special technique of the basic movement form clearing and supporting) and named as basic Parkour techniques and disseminated via the Internet.

This is sometimes rather confusing, for the basic moves and a few selected techniques are often listed without any apparent structure and may also be written in several languages.

The same is true for Freerunning. By considering Parkour techniques as basic Freerunning techniques, and the creative and acrobatic moves as advanced techniques, we can form some sort of structure.

The table below shows the abundance of terms for Parkour and Freerunning techniques. The numbers in brackets indicate the sources that have named the respective terms. We have tried to group the techniques into categories. The terms in bold represent the basic moves, as much as possible, without adding terms. The normal typeface elements are special techniques and variants of these techniques.

Table 4: Moves described as Parkour and Freerunning techniques from five different sources.

French	English
1 **Equilibre (5)**	**Balance (4,5)** Cat Balance (4) Handstand (4)
2 Quadrupédie (3)	Cat Walking (3)
3 Saut à l'arrêt (3) Saut de détente (1,2)/ Saut d'élan (2) Saut de fond (1,2) Saut de précision (1,2,3) Tic-Tac (1,5)/ Tic-Tac (2,3)	Standing Jump/s (3/5) Running Jumps (5) Drop Jumps (5) Dismount (4) Forward Drop (5) Precision (3) Standing Precision Jump (5) Precision – 1 foot (4) Precision – 2 foot (4) Running Precision (4) Tic-Tac (3) Tic-Tac (4) Stepping Movements (5) Tic-Tac To-Cat (4) Tic-Tac To-Crane (4) Tic-Tac To-Precision (4) 360° Tic-Tac (5)
4 **Réception (2,3)**	**Landing (3)** **Landing Basics (5)** Straight Landing (5) Staggered Landing (5) Crane (4)/Crane Jump (5) Crane Moonstep (4) Landing from a Drop (4)
5 **Roulade (1,3,5)**	Roll (4), Rolling (3), Rolls (5) Diving Roll (4)
6 **Passe barrière (2)/ passement (1,2,3,5)**	**Vaults (5)** Step Vault (5) Lazy Vault (3,4) Lateral Vault (5)

French	English
	"Slide Monkey" Vault (5)
Saut de chat (1,2,5)/	Kong Vault (4,5)/
passement de chat (3)	Cat Path (3)/Monkey (5)
	Kong To Precision (4)
	Kong To Cat (4)
	Diving Kong (4)
	Double Kong Vault (4)
Passement speed (3)	Speed Vault (3,4)
Passement assis (3)	Dash Vault (3,4)
	Kash Vault (4)
Réverse (1)/	Reverse (3)/
Passement arrière (3)	Reverse Vault (4)
Demi-tour (1,2)	Turn Vault (4,5)
	Palm Spin (4)

	French	English
7	Grimper (1)	**Climbing (5)**
		Mounts (5)
		Pop-Vault (5)
		Corkscrew Pop-up (5)
	Petit passe muraille (3)	Small Wall-up (3)/
		Wallhop (4)
	Passe muraille (1,2,3,5)	Wall-up (3)/Wall Run (4)/
		Wall Run (5)
	360° passe muraille (3)	360° Wall-up (3)/
		360° Wallhop (4)
	Planche (1,2)	
	Saut de bras (1,2,3,5)	Arm Jumps (5)/
		Cat Leap (3,4)
		Running Cat Leap (4)
		Level To Level Cat (4)
	Retour de bras (5)	Cat-to-Cat (5)
		180° Cat (4)
		270° Cat (4)
		360° Cat (4)

	French	English
8	Laché (1,2,5)	**Swings and Hanging Movements (5)**
	Montée de bras (5)	Dyno (5)
		Straight Laché (5)
		Swinging Laché (5)
	Le balancer (2)	

	French	English
9	Franchissement (1,2,5)	Underbar (4,5)/Clearing (5) Spiral Underbar (5) Feet-First Underbar (5)
10		Aerial (4) Back flip (4)
11		Wall Spin (4)
12		Flag (4)

Sources:

1 = Kalteis, A. & Meyer, D. (Parkour Grundbewegungen) – Internet source

2 = Parkour Association Germany (Parkour – Techniques) – Internet source

3 = Sébastien, F. (Freerunning Techniques) – Internet source

4 = Urban Free Flow (Parkour/Freerun Techniques) – Internet source

5 = Edwards, D. (The Parkour & Freerunning Handbook) – London: Virgin Books

In this book, we have tried to divide the basic PK & FR techniques and a few selected Freerunning tricks into movement categories to formulate movement descriptions and provide methodical steps to learn these techniques.

The authors have divided the basic Parkour and Freerunning techniques as follows:

PARKOUR & FREERUNNING – BASIC MOVES
- Balancing
- Running
- Jumps
- Landings
- Vaults
- Climbing
- Hanging and swinging
- Clearing

FREERUNNING – ADVANCED MOVES
- Loops
- Wall tricks

However, there is some overlap and inaccuracy in the case of a few techniques, so we have made some modifications, for example classified the "Arm-Jump/Cat Leap – Saut de bras" in the category of climbing techniques. Close examination of this movement could reveal a landing in a hanging position followed by clearance from this hanging position. In this case, we have decided to classify it as a climbing technique because the "Arm Jump/Saut de bras" is nearly always used in order to climb up to a higher level.

The following chapter contains more detailed descriptions of the techniques and examples are provided for methodical approaches both outdoors and indoors.

4.1   BALANCING – ÉQUILIBRE

Balance plays a key role in all human movement, which is why it is at the top of our list.

In Parkour and Freerunning, good balance ability is not only an essential pre requisite, but is an essential component of training along with self-evaluation and concentration. Particularly for balancing exercises on railings, in precision jumps and at dizzying heights, it is important to be able to control your balance under tough physical and emotional conditions. For this reason, balance should be trained regularly.

Balance means using muscle strength to keep the body upright against the forces of gravity by positioning the body's center of gravity over the point of support. The fewer balancing movements required, the more economical and therefore more harmonious and controlled the movements and "staying upright" (static balancing). The narrower the support surfaces (e.g., standing on tip-toes or on a railing), the harder it is for the body to balance.

Balance ability is a complex process that is determined by many factors. Firstly, visual control plays a key role, i.e. the eyes see buildings, walls or the ground, which enables our brains to control our body position in space. That is very easy to test, by standing on one leg and then closing your eyes. With your eyes closed, it is much more difficult to balance on one leg than with your eyes open. Other control systems for our position in space are situated in our inner ear.

The vestibular system is a spatial orientation organ inside the inner ear. It is composed of a series of tubes, fluids and tiny, sensitive hairs that, if, for example, the head suddenly moves by tilting, the brain helps to register it as an apparent "tilting of the whole body." This system is often called the organ of balance. However, these messages can also be misleading. Try this test: stand on one leg, close your eyes and start to circle your head. Can you stand up for more than 10 seconds?

Now do the same test with your eyes open and focus on one point. You will see that it is much easier to remain upright because the information received by the eyes has triumphed over that obtained by the vestibular system. The eyes are the most important sources of information in the human balance system.

Another control system is the kinesthetic perception in our muscles. Our muscles must constantly work together to keep our bodies balanced. One of the roles of the muscle spindles in the muscles is to give feedback to the brain on the tension ratios and therefore the angles of the limbs relative to each other. If the body leans to the side when balancing, the stretched muscles on that side of the body report that the body is not in the desired balance position.

Finally, tactile perception, for example the perception of pressure under the soles of the feet, is also important for finding and keeping balance.

Regular balance training can be done at the start of a workout, e.g., during the special warm-up phase. Balance training helps to activate the foot muscles and supporting musculature and to sharpen concentration for the workout to follow. It is a good idea to carry out specific balance training at the start of a workout as that is when concentration is still very high.

From a sports-science point of view, balance ability can be divided into:
- static balance (standing) and
- dynamic balance (movement, flight and turning balance).

4.1.1   BALANCE BASICS

A) STATIC BALANCE
Static balance ability tries to keep the body in balance without significant changes of position. Absolutely immobile static balance is impossible. An example of (almost) static balance ability is the front horizontal balance. If you watch the supporting foot (best done barefoot), you will see very clearly how hard the person has to work to keep his balance.

Training is done in different positions on narrow support surfaces, such as the one-legged stand, lying on the stomach or back, "crossways" sitting with bent knees, free-handed parallel sitting on beams and railings, Cat Balance (see page 89) on railings, slow changes of position and combinations of different positions, and, of course, handstands. The smaller and narrower the surface of the body and the apparatus, the longer the position must be held, the longer the combination of different positions is and the softer the surface, the greater the challenge and effects of the exercise.

B) DYNAMIC BALANCING: MOVEMENT, FLIGHT AND TURNING BALANCE
Dynamic balance involves three challenge situations:

1. Movement balance: During the movement, the body must "constantly seek and keep balance" in space, which becomes clear when balancing on a pole.
2. Flight balance: quick changes of position with free movements in the air can be standing jumps (from wall to wall) or also drop jumps. If your arms flail about in the air, this excess movement indicates that you are fighting to keep balance.
3. Turning balance: balance must also be kept during turns, with the aid of the arms.

Movements under time pressure and changing conditions, as is typical for Parkour runs, benefit from well-developed dynamic balance ability. Training of the dynamic balance ability can be carried out by the repeated practice of Parkour-specific basic movement forms under difficult, innovative and tricky balance conditions. Rapid transitions from standing to sitting or kneeling may also be included.

Additional vestibular stimuli in the inner ear are triggered by rotation, which is an additional complication. Turning around the longitudinal axis or rolling (page 126), handstands (page 90) and somersaults (page 221) are some of these more complicated movement situations that should be practiced frequently.

C) COMBINATIONS OF DYNAMIC AND STATIC BALANCING MOVES:
REGAINING A STATE OF (NEAR) STATIC BALANCE

Regaining balance when coming out of a movement is a combination that can mainly be seen when performing a standing landing after a jump. Coming to a stop on a narrow beam after running and standing on one leg for 2-3 seconds; jumping, then landing on one leg, and drop jumps from walls to a standstill are examples of this third group.

In Parkour, there are three types of balance tasks: balancing on the feet, on all fours and on the hands.

4.1.2   BALANCING ON THE FEET

In PK & FR, good balancing skills means being able to move under control on different surfaces and at different heights. Narrow walls, railings and branches may represent special challenges to the balance abilities.

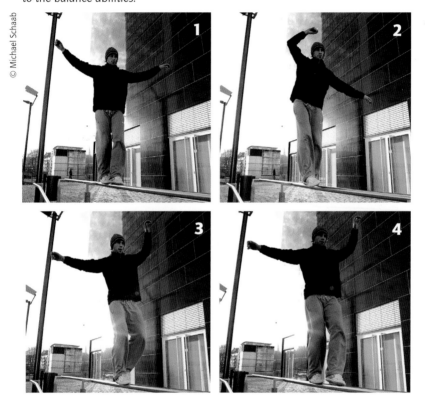

Photo sequence

1: balance

Balancing on the feet can be practiced almost anywhere. Beginners can start with standing balance, trying to keep balance on one leg. This simple exercise can be made more difficult by adding specific movements of the free leg or head. Closing the eyes when standing on one leg is already quite a challenge for most people.

Dynamic balance exercises on the feet should be practiced regularly on different surfaces and at different heights. Suitable locations are narrow walls, railings and poles in the most different executions. It is important to increase the difficulty gradually, particularly the height.

Bear in mind the motto, "don't take unnecessary risks." If you are doing balance training at heights, in order to work on your concentration, you should never practice at a height you are not comfortable jumping down from. Kids' playgrounds are good places to practice your balance on railings, and the ground is often covered with sand or some other soft surface.

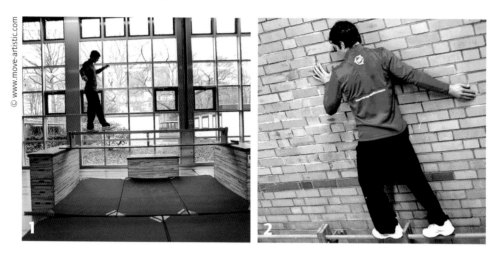

© www.move-artistic.com

Balance – ways of using apparatus in the gym

4.1.3   CAT BALANCE (BALANCING ON ALL FOURS)

The term Cat Balance is used for balancing on all fours. This technique is particularly suited to climbing up steep walls when it is only possible to balance on the balls of the feet and it would

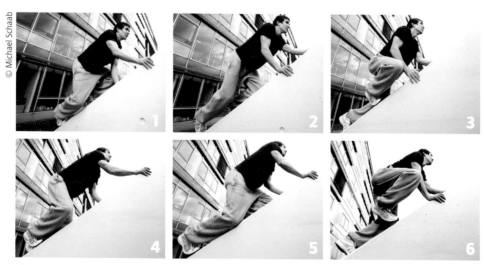

© Michael Schaab

Photo sequence 2: Cat Balance

therefore be hard to balance without using the hands to provide additional stability. Balancing on all fours is also facilitated by a lowered center of gravity.

MOVEMENT DESCRIPTION:

The Cat Balance involves balancing on your hands and the balls of your feet. It is a good idea to keep your hips and center of gravity as close as possible to the obstacle (narrow wall or railing) so that your knees fall on either side of the obstacle. Look in your direction of movement and move your hands and feet alternately in the direction of movement.

Balancing on all fours can, like all balancing exercises, first be practiced on the floor. You can just use a line drawn on the floor along which you move on all fours. Make it harder by perfecting the action along narrow, hip-height walls. The hardest place to perform the Cat Balance is on a railing that not only challenges your balance ability to the limit but also requires sufficient hand and lower arm strength. Difficulty and height should be increased gradually.

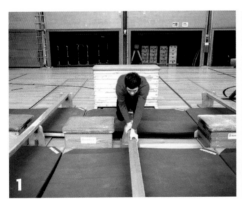 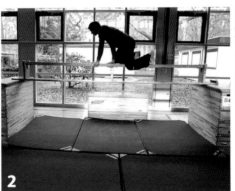

© www.move-artistic.com

Cat Balance – examples for apparatus in a gym

4.1.3   HANDSTAND (BALANCING ON THE HANDS)

In PK & FR videos, handstands are shown in many different locations: on walls, on railings, on roofs at dizzying heights, etc.

Before learning how to go up into a handstand, first gain experience of the basic requirements, such as *body support, tension and spatial orientation ability when upside-down* and then with the handstand itself, with help.

Swinging the legs up and lifting them up into a handstand brings additional coordination tasks and great challenges for the balance abilities on the hands.

© Adalm Lachner Photography

Ábel Kocsis – Handstand in Budapest

MOVEMENT DESCRIPTION:

Preparation

- From a standing position, raise the hands above the head as an extension of the torso as they will be deployed in the handstand position. Take a long step forward onto the base leg in a long lunge.
- Weight on the front, load-bearing base leg, arms still held in line with the torso.
- Lower the upper body forward.
- Place the hands shoulder-width apart, keeping the arms in line with the torso. Bend the knees and hips while swinging the free leg up and back.

Execution

- The free leg swings vertically up and back, while the base leg straightens due to the pulling of the free leg.
- Bring your center of gravity over the support point keeping your body extended (don't hollow your back!), keeping your seat (center of gravity) over your hands (support point). The legs complete the handstand. The head is kept in line with the torso and the eyes look at the floor.

Landing

- Lower the base leg (the first "landing leg") near the hands and lift/push off the hands from the floor.
- Raise the upper body and place the second foot (previously the base leg) on the floor in a lunge position behind the body.
- Transfer body weight to the rear leg.

Basic Spotting:

When swinging up into the handstand, 1-2 spotters stand **in front of** the athlete and each holds their nearest hand against the athlete's thighs to lift him prematurely. The hand farthest away clasps the vertical thigh to support (overhand grip) and stop him from falling over. This spotting grip then acts as a balancing aid and the novice handstander can also use it as a way of supporting his body to stop his arms from giving way.

METHODOLOGY *Outdoor/Indoor*

LEARNING STEPS:

1. Creating and checking the prerequisites

a) Perform several quick tuck handstands, one after the other.

b) Hold body tension exercises:

>   **1.** Consciously hold body tension in the back (contract the buttock muscles and the long back extensors): lie on your back and contract all muscles. A partner lifts the feet of the athlete lying down from the floor, who remains as stiff as a board. **Variation:** get up out of the push-up position onto the back (with the back on the floor).
>
>   **2.** Lying on your back, and without hollowing your back, raise your arms and legs slightly from the floor.
>
>   **3.** Perform the same exercise lying on your stomach.
>
>   **4.** Stand on the balls of your feet with your arms raised in line with your body and with tensed body posture.

c) Hold the push-up position while looking at the floor:

>   **1.** Push up looking at the floor: consciously hold body tension in the front of the body (quadriceps, hip flexors and abdominal muscles) in combination with the correct support behavior. The athlete adopts the push-up position and is checked over by the partner (focus on contraction in the supporting muscle groups – see above). Then the athlete's feet are raised from the floor slightly above horizontal and he must retain the extended body posture.
>
>   **2.** From a standing position with body tension supported diagonally against a wall, push-up. Hands are slightly raised.
>
>   **3.** Hold the push-up position on the floor.
>
>   **4.** Push-up position, feet are resting on a slightly raised object whose height is gradually increased.

2. Push-up against the wall/wall handstand

Target: Keep the tensed body above the head under simplified conditions.

Task: Push up against the wall: wall handstand. From a tuck handstand position with your back to the wall, climb up the wall with your feet to reach a full handstand position, briefly remaining in the "push-up position" against the wall. A partner, standing to the side, gives verbal and physical feedback as to whether the body is straight or not (Buttock muscles tensed? Hollow back? Legs bent?).

3. Vertical wall handstand assisted by partner

Target: Incorporating handstand-specific postural features

Task: Starting from a tuck handstand position with your back against the wall, take a long step up into the wall handstand. A partner holds your thigh and raises you away from the wall into a vertical handstand. Check postural features in two or three performances of the exercise (see below):

- Is the abdomen pulled in (no hollow back)?
- Are the buttocks tensed (check for contraction – the contraction of the buttocks must cause the trousers to crease!)?
- Is the head in line with the body? (Do not tuck the head into the back of the neck or forward onto the chest but look at the floor.)
- Is the arm-torso angle extended? (Consciously check again: place your back against the wall/box and hold your arms stretched above your head: do your arms touch the wall/box?)
- Do you stretch your shoulders out to the ceiling? (Narrow the shoulders instead of stretching them wide. Try this out first in a standing position. Sit with your arms up against the resistance of a partner's hands, lean on them, pushing your hands to the ceiling.) The helpers can pull you from the floor by the shoulders to provide support.

4. Swinging up into the handstand assisted by a partner or against the wall, then lowering from the handstand down to a standing position

Target: Learn to go up into a handstand and how to come out of a handstand in a controlled manner.

Task: From a standing position, raise the arms and step forward into a long lunge step, transferring your bodyweight onto the front base leg. Swing up to a sloping handstand. Lower and straighten up into the lunge by raising your arms, then lower them again and swing up into an extended handstand. A partner helps you to keep balance by holding your thigh. Spread out your legs into a straddle position keeping your center of gravity high (i.e., keep your buttocks up for a long time!), slowly lower down into the lunge position and then stand up straight.

Variations: swing up to the handstand from different surfaces and in different physical situations (e.g., from raised surfaces).

Different ways of coming into the handstand: From a half-tuck position, lean onto your hands and jump to go up into a handstand. Advanced athletes can also go up into a handstand in slow motion. For this, the shoulders must first be shifted over the hands, then the buttocks over the head and the support point, and the legs should only be raised last.

4.2 RUNNING – COURIR

Everything in Parkour and Freerunning starts with running and sprinting, so they should always be included in training. In addition, most techniques are preceded by a short approach or a quick acceleration.

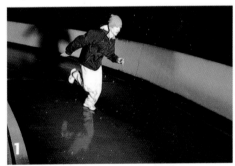 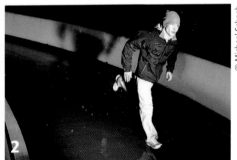

© Michael Schaab

Running

A special feature of running in PK and FR is the clearing of obstacles. This action, like all running and sprinting techniques, is characterized by a landing phase with a direct take-off phase (stretch-shortening cycle, see pages 41, 56). One first really becomes aware of these movement phases when, while striding over narrow obstacles, a precise landing is required. During the direct take-off, one must calculate the exact distance and height of the jump.

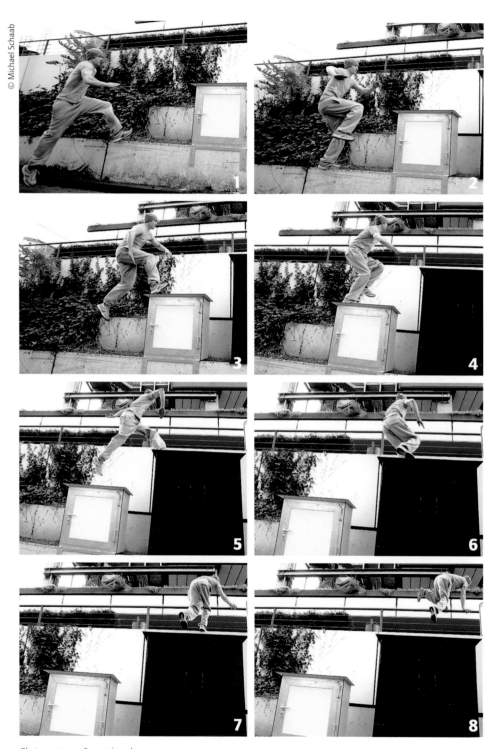

© Michael Schaab

Photo sequence 3: running clearance

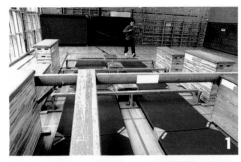

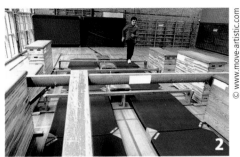

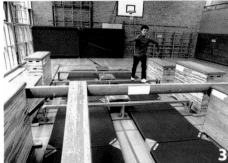

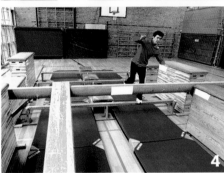

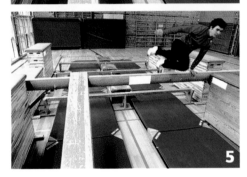

© www.move-artistic.com

Running clearance – example of an apparatus layout in a gym

According to our experience, training involves many short runs. This is because most people train in places where the spatial or architectural features seem interesting, and where individual techniques or short runs with technique combinations are practiced. This means that one often only runs at a moderate speed and that the techniques are preceded by short, quick accelerations.

Although the movements in PK & FR usually have a high-speed strength component, and endurance does not seem to be particularly solicited, we recommend that beginners start with **regular jogging training** in order to build a **general endurance base** (see Chapter 3.2.2, page 54 onward). As well as health-promoting effects, such as the prevention of cardiovascular diseases, the stabilizing of the immune system and increased mental resilience, good basic endurance above all **delays the onset of fatigue** during workouts and enables a **faster recovery between the short, quick accelerations and at the end of the training load**. For this reason, regular basic endurance training is also recommended for advanced practitioners.

4.3   JUMPS – DES SAUTS

Jumps are used to overcome **height differences, jump over gaps and obstacles,** or **jump into limited spaces**. There are numerous different jump forms that are adapted to the selected path and obstacles. Most movement techniques in PK & FR are introduced by take-offs. The jumps or take-offs can be performed from two or one legs or from a lunge position, from a standing position or a running start.

Jumps are an essential part of every PK & FR workout and are a good way to optimize and strengthen the interaction of the muscles of the lower extremities (foot, lower leg, thigh and gluteal muscles). However, as jumps are in most cases relatively taxing for the body, they should only be performed when well warmed up.

The illustration below shows an overview of selected jump forms in PK & FR.

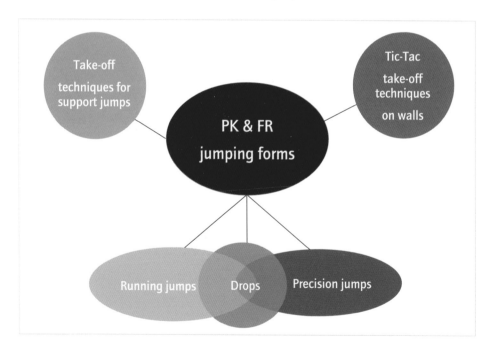

Fig. 12: Simplified representation of different jumping forms in PK & FR

As well as familiar jumping forms that are also used in other sports, there are a few special jump techniques that have gained in popularity since the emergence of PK & FR. These are explained in more detail below. Any jumping form is inextricably linked with a landing, and the two should always be considered together as a unit.

4.3.1 TAKE-OFF TECHNIQUES FOR SUPPORT JUMPS

There are three different take-off techniques for support jumps:

- One-footed take-offs (page 106)
- Two-footed take-offs (page 108)
- Take-offs from the lunge position (page 110)

One can go for different take-off techniques depending on the clearance technique used, approach possibilities and approach speed. For *one-footed* take-offs, the opposing leg is usually used as a free leg in order to raise the hips (center of gravity) over the obstacle.

Two-footed take-offs are often started from a standing position, as greater height can be achieved with a two-footed take-off. The take-off action for two-footed take-offs on the run resembles a bounce jump.

A favorite running take-off is a take-off from the lunge position. This technique is chosen in the "Kong Vault – Saut de Chat" (page 144 onward) on hard surfaces. The feet are placed one in front of the other in a lunge position. In the take-off, the front foot is last to leave the ground. The arms are swung through from behind, around the sides and then forward toward the support point to support the action.

4.3.2 TIC-TAC – STEPPING MOVEMENTS

The term *stepping movements* describes all movements that involve **pushing off from a wall**. The classic example is a Tic-Tac, which is described in more detail in this chapter.

Tic-Tac is the term for **pushing off a wall with the balls of the feet** in order to gain *height*. In principle, the Tic-Tac is a take-off from the wall, which is why we have grouped this technique with the jumps.

Usually, the Tic-Tac is combined with other techniques, such as a jump to a higher wall edge (Cat Leap – saut de chat, see page 186), a clearance technique or a precision jump.

Further examples of stepping techniques are the foot push-off during wall run, wall hop, wall flip and the push-off with the feet in the Cat-to-Cat. However, the main criterion for these movement techniques is not the push-off from the wall, which is why these techniques are not described in this chapter.

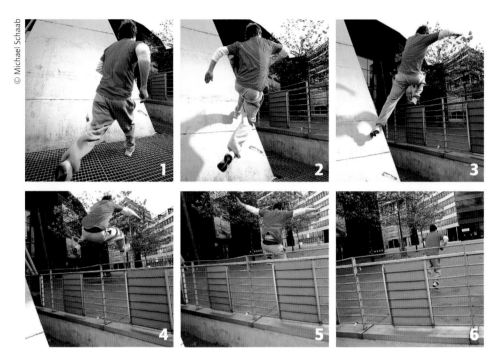

© Michael Schaab

Photo sequence 4: Tic-Tac

MOVEMENT DESCRIPTION:

Preparation

1. *Diagonal to head-on approach toward the wall (about 45°). Take-off from the floor with the leg farthest from the wall in the direction of the wall. The opposing leg nearest the wall is used as a free leg and is placed as high up the wall as possible.*

Execution

2. *The free leg near the wall touches the wall at knee to hip height with the ball of the foot (thus becoming a take-off leg), in order to push off explosively up and off the wall.*

3./4. *The knee of the free leg farther from the wall is actively pulled upward in order to gain more height and to guarantee a stable flight path. The upper body remains upright and almost parallel to the wall.*

Landing

5./6. *The ensuing landing can vary greatly for the Tic-Tac is often combined with another technique, such as a clearance technique, an arm jump/cat leap or a precision landing. If the Tic-Tac is used in order to jump over an obstacle, the landing is usually two-footed due to the increased flight phase.*

TIPS AND TRICKS

- *Place the last stride before the wall not very far away from the wall so that you do not jump against the wall.*
- *A too-close take-off is not advisable either because then there is not enough room to place the foot high enough against the wall and maintain the momentum optimally.*

Variations

1. *For this, both feet are placed one after the other while the body simultaneously turns araound its longitudinal axis. The second foot to touch the wall is used as a speed-strength push-off. The hands can also be used as support on the wall (see Tic-Tac with 180° turn on the wall example for an apparatus layout in the gym, page 104).*

Nothing is impossible

- Run with four steps around a wall corner. Two steps are placed on each wall.

METHODOLOGY

Warming up

- Practice running one-footed take-off movements for distance (e.g., running jumps).
- Practice running one-footed take-offs from low objects (curbs, tree trunks lying on the ground, etc.).

A OUTDOORS

LEARNING STEPS:

1. *From a short approach, perform a one-footed take-off from a low object, such as a curb or a knee-high wall edge.*
2. *From a short, diagonal approach, one-footed push-off from a sloping wall. Practice both with your strong and weak legs.*
3. *From a head-on approach, take two steps against the wall in order to be able to reach your outstretched hand as high as possible. Make sure your landing is controlled!*
4. *From a short, diagonal approach, one-footed push-off/take-off from a vertical wall (Tic-Tac – one wall contact) in order to gain height. Try out Tic-Tacs with your strong and weak legs.*
5. *Tic-Tac with precision landing (e.g., mark on the floor).*

6. *Tic-Tac with support of a wall or a railing.*

7. *Tic-Tac with precision landing on a wall or railing.*

8. *Tic-Tac with jump over a wall or a railing.*

9. *Tic-Tac to Cat Leap (with arm jump to follow) on the edge of a wall.*

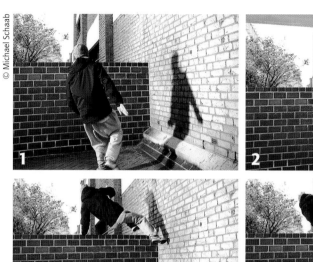

Photo sequence 5: Tic-Tac to Vault

B. INDOORS

LEARNING STEPS:

1. *From a short diagonal approach, push-off/take-off in front of a slope in order to gain height. Experiment with pushing off/taking off from the slope with your strong and weak legs.*

Layout: lean a springboard against a wall with the wide end of the springboard on the floor. Place small mats on the floor for safety.

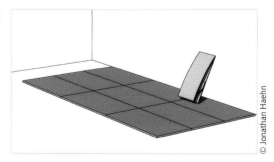

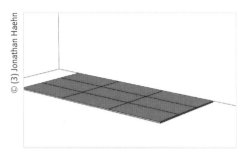

© (3) Jonathan Haehn

2. From a short diagonal approach, push/ take off from a vertical wall (Tic-Tac) to gain height. Experiment with push/take-offs from the wall with your strong and weak legs.

Layout: Place small mats near the wall for safety.

3. Tic-Tac from a diagonal approach with precision landing. The landing surface for the precision landing can be marked with a chalked circle or small mat. The landing surfaces can be varied so that the one-footed take-off from the wall (Tic-Tac) must be adapted to the direction and distance of the landing surface.

4. Tic-Tac from a diagonal approach with one-handed support on a box. The hand nearest the box is placed on it. Speed-strength take-off upward from the foot near the wall (Tic-Tac) to enable the hips to clear the box.

Layout: Place the narrow side of a long box against a wall. Place small mats behind the box for safety.

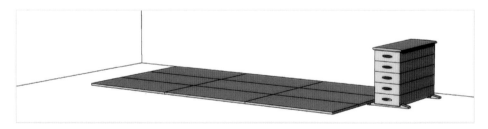

5. Tic-Tac from a diagonal approach with precision landing on the box (without using the hands).

Layout: Place the narrow side of a long box against a wall. Lay small mats in front of and behind the box for safety.

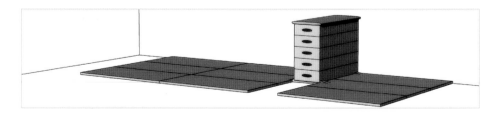

Spotter's position: Clasp the athlete's hand and forearm in order to accompany the action and to allow him to stabilize himself in the flight and landing phases.

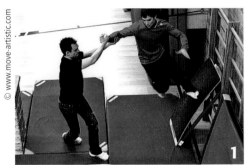 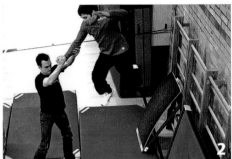

Tic-Tac to Precision

6. *Target form: Tic-Tac from a diagonal approach with a jump over the box without touching with the hands.*

Layout: See 4 (left page).

ERROR CORRECTION

Observation	Cause	Corrective Actions
The athlete slips from the wall.	The center of gravity is too close to the wall	Push away and up from the wall with the balls of the feet.
The athlete cannot gain height.	Low approach speed	Accelerate without slowing down in front of the wall. Continually increase approach speed until take-off from the wall.
	Free leg hangs down during push-off from wall	Tuck the free leg up in order to gain height.
	Fear	First, complete many reps on a sloping board, then place the board more steeply.
	Too loose in the hips	Hop on left and right feet, briefly holding the tucked up free leg.

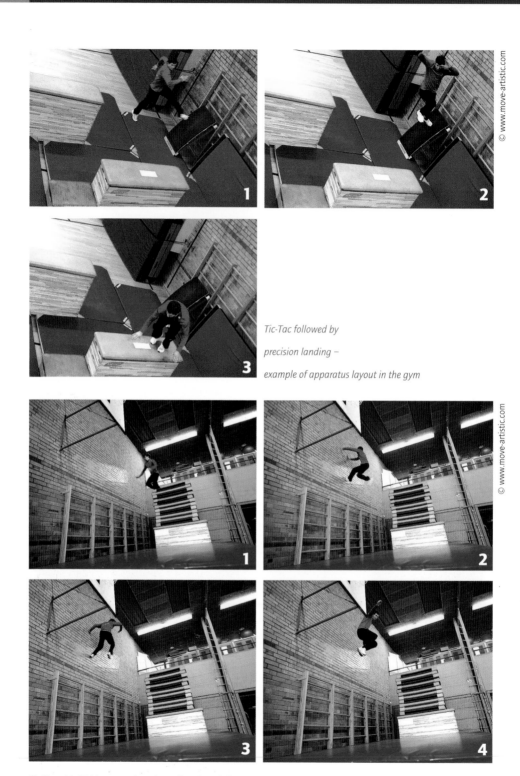

Tic-Tac followed by

precision landing –

example of apparatus layout in the gym

Tic-Tac with 180° turn against the wall – example for an apparatus layout in the gym (for advanced traceurs).

4.3.3 PRECISION JUMPS – DES SAUTS DE PRÉCISION

Precision jumps are an important element in urban displacement and should be practiced in various forms. They are characterized by an extremely precise landing, e.g., on a small wall surface or railings. Such jumps always require concentration and an awareness of one's own limitations. They require courage and confidence in one's own physical abilities.

Basically, there are three different types of precision jump:

1. One-footed (from standing)
2. Two-footed (from standing)
3. Running.

It is important to first practice these precision jumps near the floor and to increase the difficulty gradually.

TIP

If after extensive practice you dare to perform precision jumps and landings from certain heights, you should always have a "plan B" lined up in case you tumble forward or fall back while landing. Even experienced traceurs and freerunners may still make mistakes.

© www.move-artistic.com

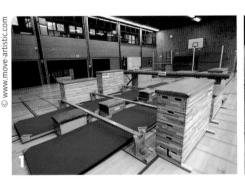
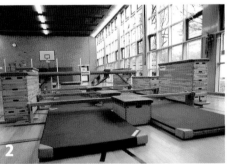

Examples for apparatus layouts
in the gym

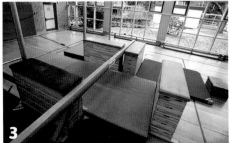

4.3.3.1   ONE-FOOT PRECISION

The *one-foot precision* is one of the easiest moves and is best suited to **small gaps**, especially if the landing surface for the precision landing is lower than the take-off. This technique is often taught first as an introduction to precision jumps for beginners.

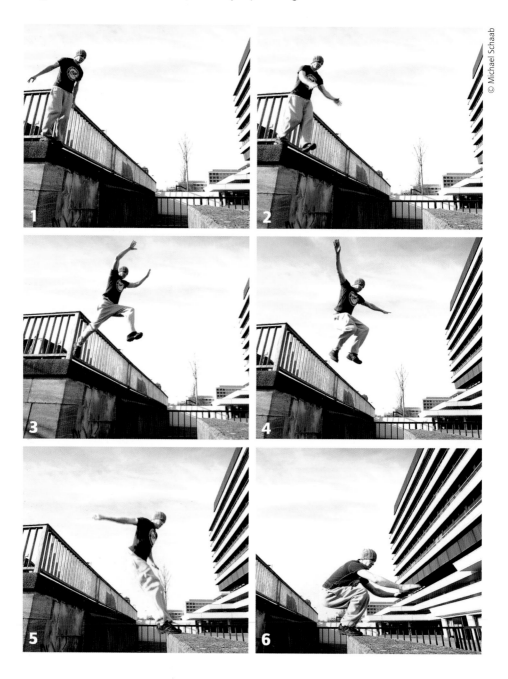

© Michael Schaab

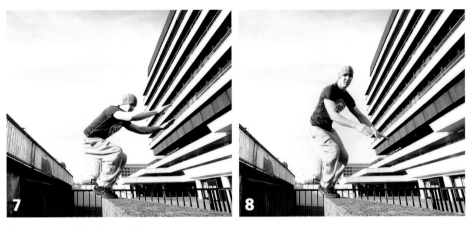

Photo sequence 6: One-foot precision

The free leg is used to target the landing surface. During the flight phase, the legs are brought parallel to each other again so that *both feet land at the same time*.

The disadvantage of this variation is that it does not allow you to jump very far.

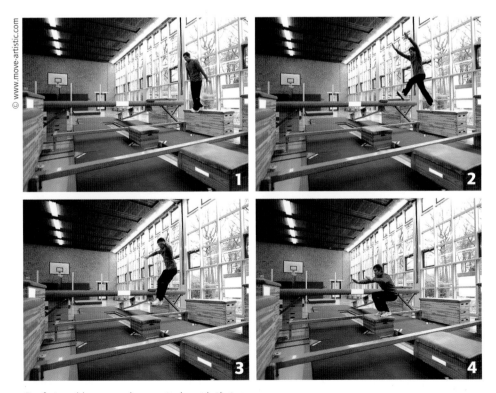

One-foot precision – example apparatus layout in the gym

4.3.3.2   TWO-FOOT PRECISION

With the *two-foot precision*, one can **jump a lot farther** than with the one-foot precision, but it does require more practice.

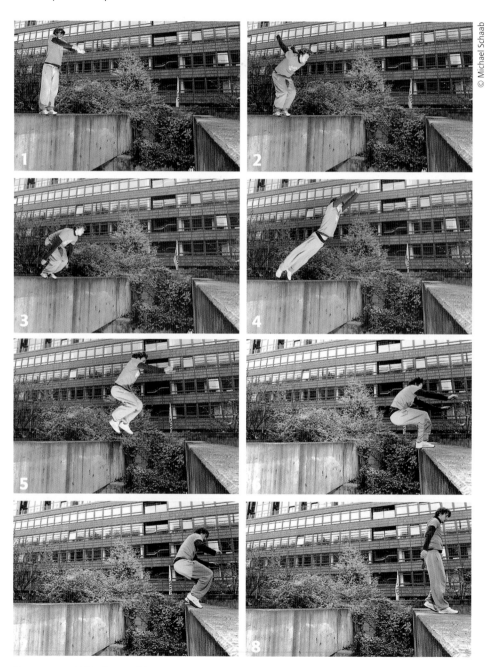

Photo sequence 7: Two-foot precision

This jump technique is characterized by a *two-foot take-off* and a *two-foot landing*. The arms are used to give momentum and swing forward and upward at the sides of the body. The landing of the precision jump is usually on the balls of the feet to ensure better and quicker balance control. If one lands on the center of the foot, there is a danger of slipping off the landing surface and falling on your butt or back, particularly when landing on railings or narrow surfaces.

© www.move-artistic.com

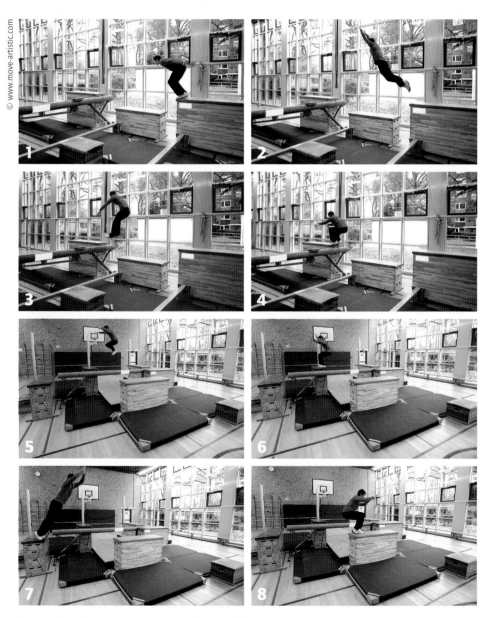

Two-footed precision jump – example apparatus layout in the gym

4.3.3.3 RUNNING PRECISION

Running precision jumps are common. Take-off is from one foot on the run, and the landing is on both feet (balls of the feet). This technique allows for clearance of the **greatest distances**. However, the greater the distance, the harder it is to achieve a precise landing.

© Michael Schaab

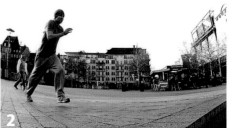

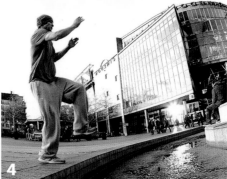

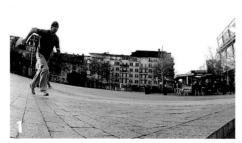

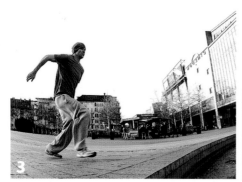

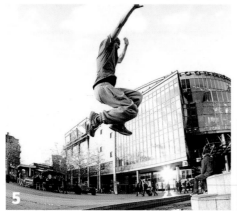

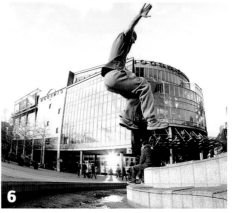

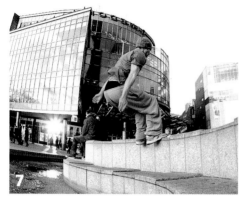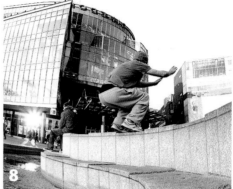

Photo sequence 8: Running precision jump

TIP

To make the landing easier, jump in a high flight curve so that you land more from above and do not have to compensate for too much forward momentum when landing.

Outdoors, one inevitably practices all precision jump variations. Indoors one can set up precision jumps so that beginners can learn and practice them separately.

© www.move-artistic.com

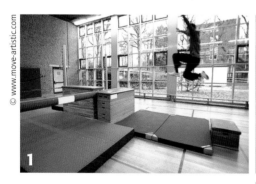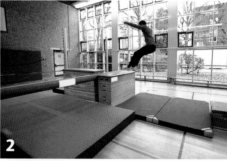

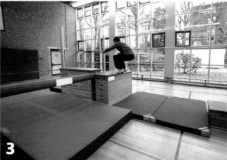

Running Precision –

Example apparatus layout in the gym

4.3.4 DROPS – SAUTS DE FOND

A *drop* is an active jump from a higher to a lower level.

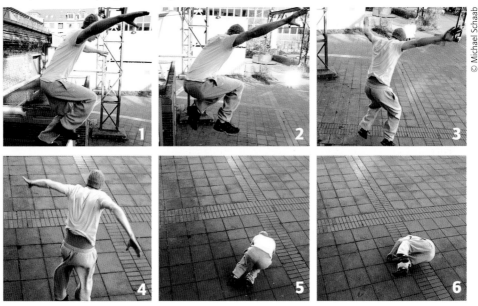

Photo sequence 9: Drop

No special skill is needed for the take-off, just don't jump too high, otherwise the landing will be harder. It is important to decide the type of landing **before** take-off, as a good landing preparation starts at take-off. Another feature of drops is a long flight path. In order to maintain control during the flight phase, it is important to **keep your head up** and to **keep your eyes on the landing spot** to avoid leaning forward too much while in the air. High drops are followed by a roll on landing when possible.

In training, drops should only be tried very gradually and practiced regularly due to the relatively high stress they place on the body and the joints.

Regular drop training (up to a maximal height of 2.2 yards) should only be undertaken by professionals.

TIPS

*We advise beginners to always practice on a soft surface or mats. Even for advanced practitioners, we do not advise doing **drops above head-height** onto a hard surface. This is just a rough guideline though as the resilience of physical structures is dependent upon age/ability, gender, fitness and previous injuries.*

4.4   LANDING BASICS – RÉCEPTION

"What goes up must come down..."

Every jump is followed by a landing. PK & FR involve running over different obstacles, moving between different levels in the process. This is why the inseparable pair of jumps and landings is one of the basic techniques of this discipline.

For this reason, even beginners should integrate a varied landing training into their learning, practicing and training.

In Parkour, the choice of **landing strategy** is firstly dependent upon:

- The *preceding technique* and secondly upon
- The *type of landing surface*.

Furthermore, landings should be adapted to:

- the *take-off height* and
- the *distance*

of the jump.

Parkour is all about continuous forward motion, which means that landing strategies are different than for example in gymnastics, where landings should be as immobile as possible.

Parkour also involves treating one's own body very responsibly so that the preference is for as controlled and soft a landing as possible.

Figure 13[1] shows an overview of the different landing strategies in PK & FR. In this book, we differentiate between **one-footed** and **two-footed landings**. While **one-footed landings** are used only **between similar levels** and **small height differences**, two-footed landings are used on **similar levels** and for drops to **a lot deeper levels**.

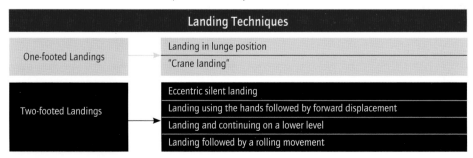

Fig. 13: Overview of landing techniques in PK & FR (foot landings)

---
1   Scientific findings of three different landing techniques can be found in Appendix 2, pp. 312-319.

4.4.1 ONE-FOOTED LANDINGS

One-footed landings are usually performed after jumps **on the same level** or with **small** height differences.

In this chapter, we will describe two one-footed landing techniques in detail.

4.4.1.1 LANDING IN THE LUNGE POSITION

A so-called *landing in the lunge position* is used after support jumps in order to be able to jog away directly after landing. You land first on one foot, then the second foot is planted afterward in the lunge position to enable you to jog off smoothly right away.

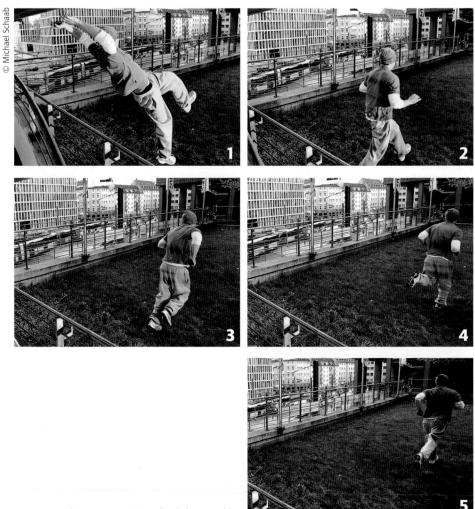

© Michael Schaab

Photo sequence 10: Landing in lunge position

4.4.1.2   CRANE

The Crane is a special landing technique that is used **when a two-footed landing is impossible** due to the height difference or the distance involved. In this case, it is sometimes possible to place one foot on the obstacle and plant the other foot against the obstacle.

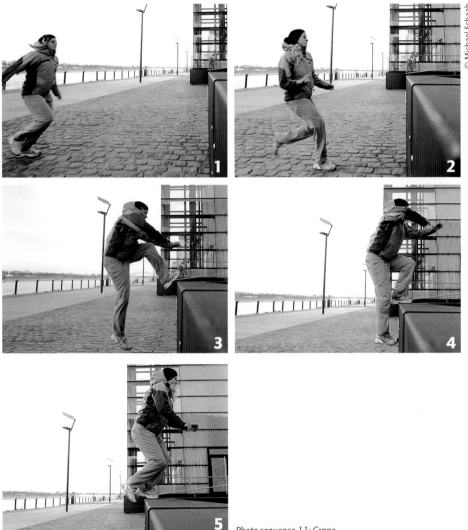

© Michael Schaab

Photo sequence 11: Crane

A Crane landing technique is also possible in precision landings when tipping backward would lead to a serious fall. A Crane landing enables a greater upper body forward lean and allows placement of the hands beside the landing foot on the landing surface for support.

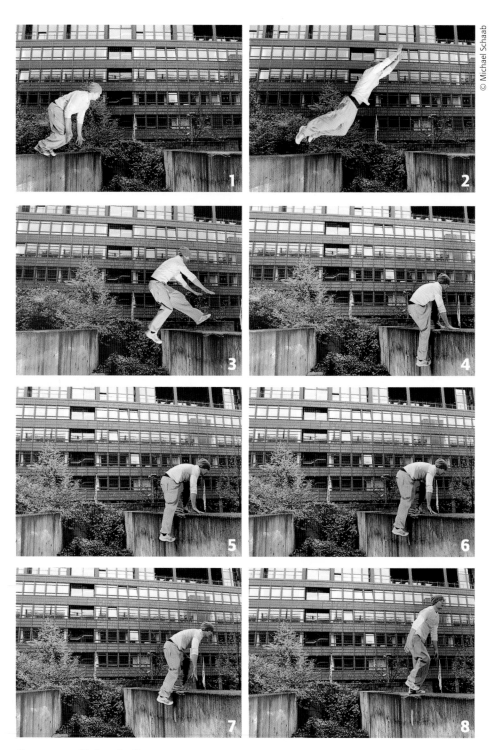

© Michael Schaab

Photo sequence 12: Crane landing

The so-called **Crane Moon Step** is a special form of the Crane landing. In this technique, the take-off foot is also the landing foot. The knee of the free leg is pulled upward and trails after the take-off leg for the landing. For the observer, this looks like a step in space, a "moon step." This technique became famous in an Urban Freeflow technique video.

In this video, the traceur runs head-on toward a wall, takes a step toward the edge of the wall followed by a moon-step and performs a Crane landing on the top of the wall. This technique allows you to climb up shoulder to head-height walls without using your hands.

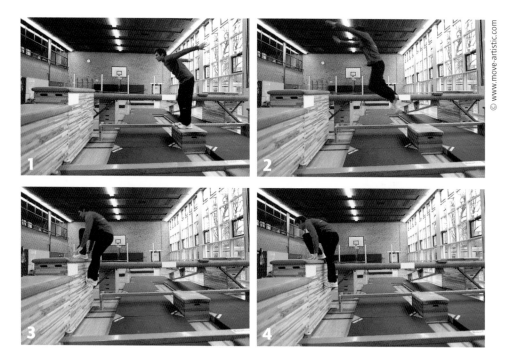

© www.move-artistic.com

Crane – example of apparatus layout in the gym

4.4.2 TWO-FOOT LANDINGS ON THE SAME LEVEL AND FOR DROPS

There are a few different forms of **two-foot landings** in Parkour and Freerunning. These landings are used both for jumps on similar levels and for drops or, to use the French term, *sauts de fond*.

There are four different basic forms of this landing:

- Two-foot, eccentric silent landing (standing)
- Two-foot landing using hands and followed by a forward movement (page 122 onward)
- Two-foot landing and continuing on a lower level (page 124 onward)
- Two-foot landing followed by roll (Parkour roll) (page 126 onward).

4.4.2.1 ECCENTRIC SILENT LANDING

In a silent landing, the aim is to absorb the body's momentum by optimal eccentric action of the ankle, knee and hip musculature. The first contact with the ground is made with the tips of the toes and the balls of the feet. The feet are roughly shoulder-width apart and are placed as parallel as possible on the floor so that the forces that act on the body during landing are divided equally down both legs.

When landing, it is particularly important that the knee-foot angles are correct, meaning the knees are always over the tips of the toes. Where the feet point, the knees follow. Bear this in mind when repeating many times during landing practice to avoid joint misalignments that can, over time, lead to joint injuries. We advise beginners to land as "softly" as possible. This focuses all your attention on the landing and guarantees an active, eccentric landing.

For drops and jumps from heights followed by silent landing, in PK & FR the hands are often placed on the ground for support. The hands can be placed on either side of the feet or between them. Whichever strategy you choose is up to you.

However, remember to make sure to put equal loading on both legs and adopt the correct knee-foot position when landing.

© Michael Schaab

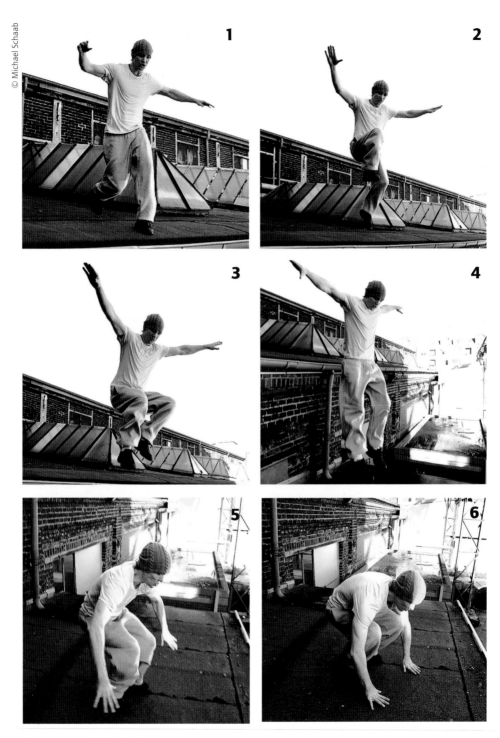

Photo sequence 13: Silent landing

STANDING PRECISION

The standing precision is a special form of two-footed silent landing. Precision landings are characterized by a **targeted landing on a small landing surface**, such as narrow walls or even railings.

Precision landings can be carried out both level to level and between different heights.

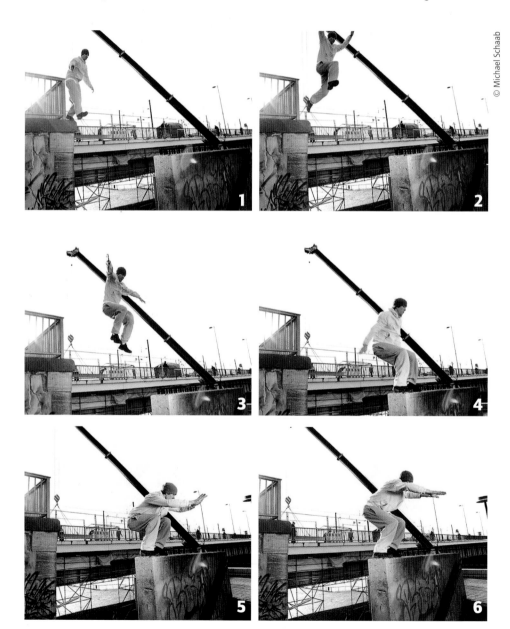

© Michael Schaab

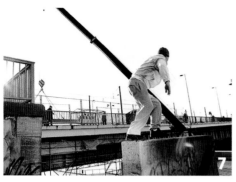
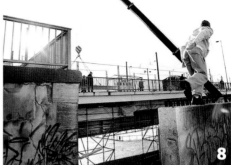

Photo sequence 14: Standing precision landing

A precision landing is landed the same way as a silent landing (toe first then heel). The smaller the landing surface, the more important is **a precise landing on the balls of the feet**, such as handrails in order to cushion the landing and control balance.

Spotting position: Precision landings can be assisted by a spotter both indoors and outdoors. The spotter's far hand holds the jumper's near hand and his other hand holds the jumper's forearm to provide additional support.

© www.move-artistic.com

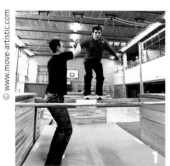
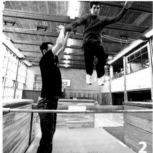
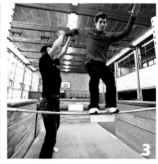

Precision jump onto a horizontal bar with partner support on the hand and forearm

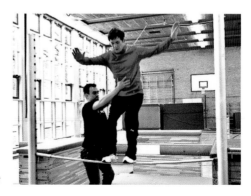

Alternative support on abdomen and back

4.4.2.2   LANDING USING THE HANDS
WITH DEVIATION TO FORWARD MOVEMENT ("LANDING AND DIVERTING")

It is possible to jog away in the jumping direction after a drop, and in Parkour and Freerunning, the hands often touch the ground to support the landing action in the case of a two-footed landing.

The hands touch the ground to allow some of the forces that act on the body during the landing to be absorbed up the arms and to allow the landing to be converted into a forward movement. This landing technique is referred to in the rest of this book as **landing and diverting**.

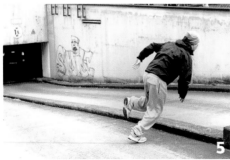
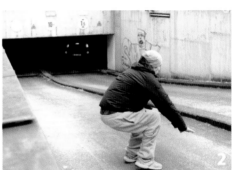
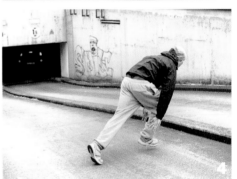
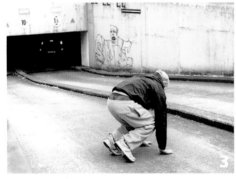
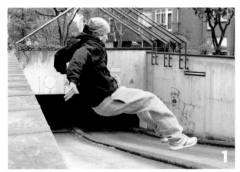

© Michael Schaab

Photo sequence 15: Landing and diverting

MOVEMENT DESCRIPTION:

Flight Phase (photo 1)

The mental preparation for a good landing starts at take-off. For drops, the body is often compact during the flight phase, i.e., the legs are tucked up. In the final phase before ground contact, the legs are stretched out to touch the ground. The tips of the toes point toward the landing surface.

Landing phase (photos 2/3)

The landing is two-footed. Ground contact is only with the forefoot and the ball of the foot. The feet are parallel and roughly shoulder-width apart. The body's momentum is optimally absorbed by the eccentric action of the ankle, knee and hip musculature. The hips are bent to such an extent that the hands can be placed in front of the feet on the ground to allow the arms to absorb some of the momentum. This body position is comparable to a sprinter's starting position.

Diversion (photos 3-5)

From this "starting block position" with the hands on the ground, the body shifts forward in the direction of movement. The aim is to jog off smoothly by pushing off from the hands and feet.

Prerequisites:

Active, eccentric silent landing for jumps from heights.

METHODOLOGY *Outdoor/Indoor*

LEARNING STEPS:

- From a standing position, go down on all fours then push up to standing position again.
- From a standing position, go down on all fours and sprint off from this position.
- On flat, surface, from a standing position or with a short approach, spring forward one or two-footed. First concentrate on a two-footed landing and then go down onto all fours and sprint off right away.
- Jump down from a low height, aiming for an active "silent" landing and then go down on all fours and "divert" the movement forward.
- Different jumps from forward movement (drops or support jumps) with two-footed landing, touching the ground with the hands then diverting the movement forward.

4.4.2.3 LANDING AND CONTINUING ONTO A LOWER LEVEL

Outdoors there are often interesting architectural features with levels at many different heights, where one can jump from a higher level such as a roof, down to a slightly lower level or a wall, and then down to the ground. In such cases, where two drop jumps are performed in a row, it is possible to land and, with the arms, transfer the momentum immediately into another drop. This is less a movement technique than a landing strategy and a way to keep the flow going when performing two drops.

If one lands in a drop with two feet on a raised object (e.g., a wall), the arms can, as in landing and diverting, be placed on the ground in front of the body and be used to transfer the momentum. In this case, the hands are not used for diversion, but more in the style of a supporting movement in order to follow with another drop.

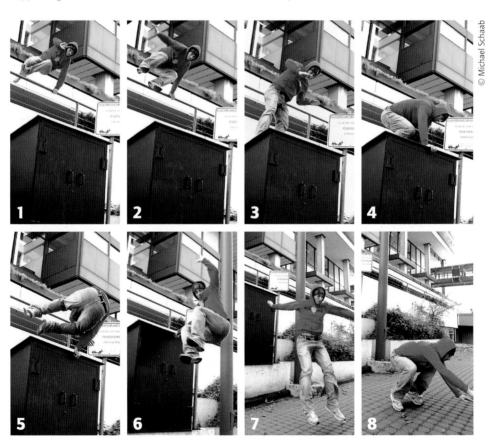

© Michael Schaab

Photo sequence 16: Landing and jogging away on a lower level

The hands can touch the ground, placed parallel in front of the body so that the transfer resembles that of a Kong vault (see indoor photo sequence below). Or put one hand down in front of the other so that the transfer resembles that of a Reverse (photo sequence 16 – landing and jogging away).

© www.move-artistic.com

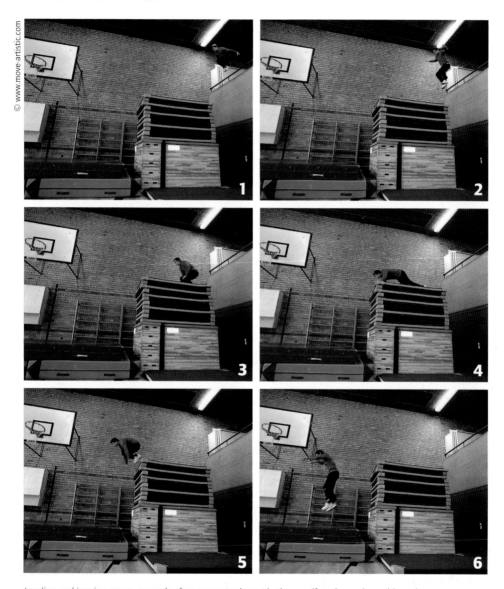

Landing and jogging away – example of an apparatus layout in the gym (for advanced practitioners)

4.4.2.4 LANDING WITH ROLL ("PK ROLL"/ROULADE)

A two-footed landing followed by a roll is a typical PK & FR landing. This landing strategy is called the PK roll, or *roulade* in French. Although these terms linguistically only describe the rolling movement, it is understood that they mean a landing followed by a roll, thus making them special landing techniques.

This landing technique is mainly used for drops from great heights or after jumps and clearance techniques with great horizontal movement speed. The purpose of the landing technique is not just to absorb and divert the body's momentum via the lower extremities, but to absorb and divert some of the momentum via the rolling movement.

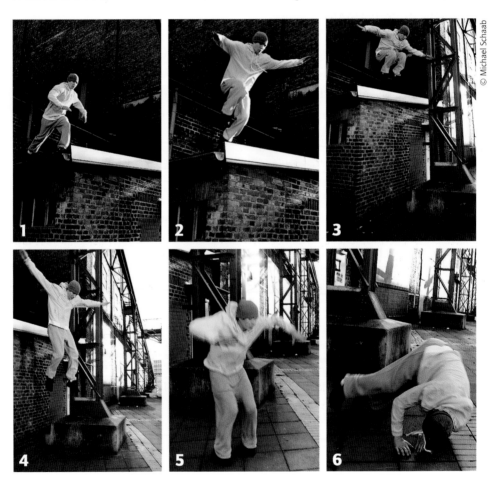

© Michael Schaab

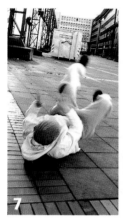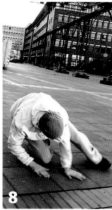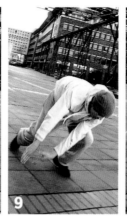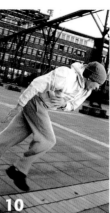

Photo sequence 17: Landing with a roll

MOVEMENT DESCRIPTION:

Flight Phase (photos 1-4)

If a jump from a great height is to be followed by a PK roll, then during the flight phase, one should bring enough horizontal energy into the movement to facilitate the diversion into the roll. In the flight phase, the legs are tucked up for compactness. To prepare for the landing, the feet are actively extended toward the ground.

Landing Phase (photo 5)

Land on the balls of the feet with the legs almost straight. The feet are parallel and roughly shoulder-width apart. The landing can be seen as a kind of conversion for going into the roll. When learning the PK roll, pay particular attention to the correct knee-foot angle (knee always above the foot) so as to avoid unfavorable joint positions and possible resulting joint damage.

Roll (photos 6-10)

Landing, diversion and roll are one movement. It is important that the feet are parallel before going into the roll. The rolling movement is diagonally over the back in order to avoid hurting the bony spine on the hard surface. Ideally, you should only roll on your back muscles because any contact of the bones with the hard surface is bound to be painful.

In order to start the roll correctly, twist the upper body and put both hands on the ground. When twisting the upper body, stick one arm out. The hand of this arm is put down before the other hand. If you roll over your right shoulder, your right hand is in front, and the left hand is in front of the right if you roll over your left shoulder. Now roll (in order) over hand, forearm, shoulder and diagonally over your back. The last part of the body to touch the ground is the side of the lumbar spine above the hips. After the roll, the body is at an angle of 45° to the starting position. The feet touch the ground, one in front of the other, ready to jog off immediately. Push up from the hands to stand up.

Prerequisites

Active, silent standing landing from jumps from higher levels (page 119).

Landing using the hands and diverting into forward motion (page 122 onwards).

METHODOLOGY *Outdoors/Indoors*

LEARNING STEPS:

- First approximation of the PK roll via forward roll, backward roll and sideways roll (on soft surface or small mats).
- First practice the rolling action diagonally across the back. The practitioner first goes down onto all fours, in a kind of push-up with the hips bent and the bottom pointing upward. Now raise one hand from the floor and place it between the opposing hand and foot. Push forward with the legs and look at the hand stretched out to the side before rolling over the forearm, shoulder and then diagonally over the back. Place the feet on the floor, one after the other, and help yourself stand up by pushing off the floor with your hands.
- Drop down to all fours from a standing position. Place the hands one in front of the other in order to simulate the upper body twist of the rolling action diagonally over the back. Push back up to a standing position.
- Drop down onto the hands placed one in front of the other and go into the rolling action diagonally over the back.
- Jump forward from level to level, landing on the balls of your feet with a silent landing and initiate the PK roll action.
- Jump down from a low height, aiming for an active landing and go into the rolling action.
- Try out different two-foot landing jumps and PK rolls, then jog away.

TIPS AND TRICKS

- *Progress gradually to trying this on hard surfaces. Before you roll on wood or stone floors, start with sand, then with forest floors and fields until your technique is fluid.*

- *If rolling on hard ground hurts the back of your hip, try to remain compact when rolling and pull more strongly to the side at the end of the roll so that you come out of the roll at a lateral angle of 90°.*

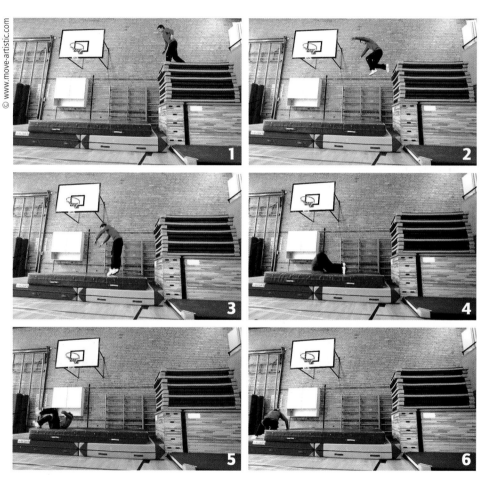

© www.move-artistic.com

Landing and rolling – example for an apparatus layout

A varied landing training on different surfaces via the regular clearance of obstacles and jumps from different heights is highly recommended even for beginners.

This kind of varied training can be combined very well with the training of precision jumps and drops.

VARIATION I: DIVING ROLL

A diving roll is comparable to a flight roll or a jump roll. The biggest difference to the flight roll is the rolling movement. As in the PK roll, roll diagonally over the back. Use the diving roll during actions such as diving across a railing.

VARIATION II: HAND SUPPORT LANDING

In Freerunning, there are a few handstand specialists who land on their hands and then push up into a handstand after a support movement such as a Kong Vault (saut de chat), (page 144). This type of landing should only be attempted with sufficient handstand experience and sufficient strength in the arms, shoulders, back and torso.

METHODOLOGY

LEARNING STEPS:

1. *Handstand*
2. *Run into a handstand*
3. *Push up into handstand (e.g., wall handstand)*
4. *First jump from standing to hands, later to handstand*
5. *Jump downward from a handstand on a mat to a handstand*

4.5   VAULTS – PASSEMENT/PASSE BARRIÈRE

To clear hip to chest-high obstacles such as walls and railings, there are many different support techniques. The choice of technique depends on the approach angle and speed and the width and height of the obstacle. The choice of support technique depends not only on the nature of the obstacle but, in many cases, is dependent upon the situation or personal preference.

In the next chapter, some typical Parkour and Freerunning techniques are described and their methodology reviewed.

© Michael Schaab

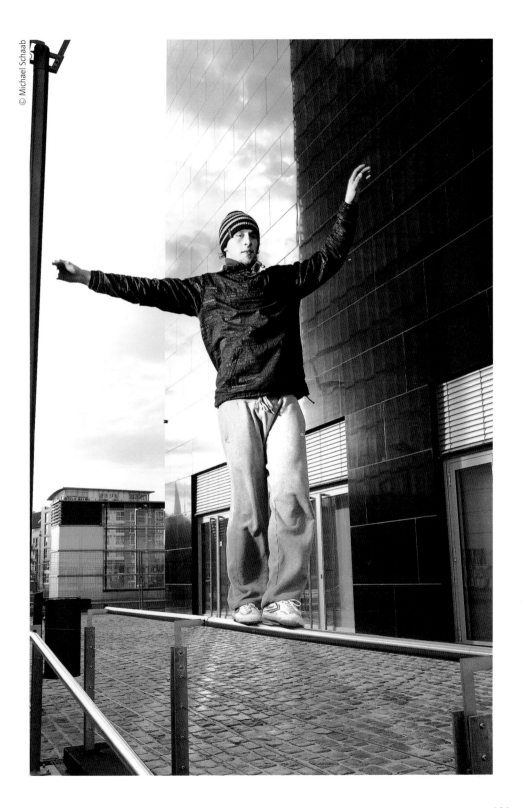

4.5.1   STEP VAULT

The Step Vault is the **easiest support technique** and a suitable foundation for most other techniques in this group. It is particularly suited to **slow approach speeds over railings** or **narrow, hip-high walls**. This technique is also appropriate when you need to concentrate on a small landing surface.

After a one-foot take-off and **support** on the obstacle, the **free leg's foot takes an intermediate step on the obstacle** (e.g., railing), while the body crosses the obstacle **without changing your angle to the obstacle**, thus being a sort of flank vault.

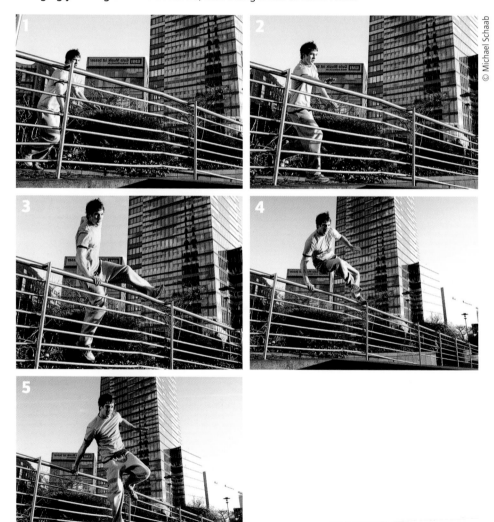

© Michael Schaab

Photo sequence 18: Step Vault

MOVEMENT DESCRIPTION:

Preparation

1. *Head-on but diagonal or side-on approach also possible.*
2. *One-footed take-off.*

Execution

3. *Both hands, or even just one, provide support on the obstacle. The rear, farther away base leg is placed to the side – not too close – next to the hands or hand on the obstacle.*
4. *The take-off leg is brought underneath the body between the hands and the supported free leg, forward over the obstacle and is first to touch the ground, without touching the obstacle.*

Landing

5. *The extended forward take-off leg is first to land. What was previously the base leg is placed in front of the landing leg (former take-off leg) so that you can jog away immediately.*

Tip: Employ a two-footed landing if there is a big height difference between the support and the landing spot.

TIPS AND TRICKS

■ *If you are already quite familiar with this technique, the approach can be accelerated. Support only with the outside hand and the free leg. Now it only takes a brief, unloaded step on the obstacle, which makes this technique appear more flowing and easy.*

METHODOLOGY   *A. Outdoors*

LEARNING STEPS:

Choose a narrow, hip-height obstacle (railing or wall).

1. *Support with both hands.*
2. *Support with one hand.*
3. *Practice on both sides: take off from your right foot and support with your right hand and your left leg, then switch sides.*
4. *Increase approach speed (possibly looking for a wider support surface).*
5. *Step Vault with drop onto a lower height/landing surface (two-footed landing).*

B. INDOORS

LEARNING STEPS:

1. *Two-footed take-off and support with both hands and lateral intermediate step on the obstacle with the free leg.*

Apparatus: Diagonally placed box with mats for safety, balance beam or hip-height horizontal bar.

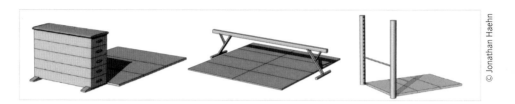

© Jonathan Haehn

2. *One-footed take-off and support with one hand and lateral intermediate step (Step Vault).*
3. *Both sides should be practiced: take-off right = support right and the same on the left side.*
4. *Increase approach speed.*
5. *Change the apparatus layout: change the height of the box, run over a vaulting horse with support or mount a horizontal bar diagonally.*

TIP FOR CHOICE OF OBSTACLE:

At increased approach speeds, it is easier to perform a step vault over a sideways box than over a horizontal bar.

4.5.2 SPEED (VAULT) – PASSEMENT RAPIDE

If you have previously tried the Step Vault, it is an easy step to the Speed Vault. As the name suggests, the Speed Vault (hereafter called *Speed*) is performed when running flat out.

The Speed can be performed in different ways:

■ At first, use the left or right arms for support.
■ Another variation is in the choice of the left or right take-off leg. This means that either the take-off leg or the free leg touches the ground first.

EXAMPLE

If you support with the left arm and take off with the left leg, then the right leg is brought to the side over the obstacle and the take-off leg is brought forward under the body so that it lands first. This clearance technique is similar to the Step Vault with just one support arm, but without an intermediate step (see photo sequence 19).

If you decide to support with the left arm, but take off with the right foot, then the left free leg must be brought over the obstacle first. In the support, the upper body bends forward and the free leg, unlike in the step vault, is brought first over the obstacle. This technique is similar to running over a hurdle with a support action and is harder to learn.

Usually, in both technique variations people have a strong and a weak side, which is why one should train both sides regularly so that the weak side is not neglected.

First we explain the more common and easier variation of the Speed in Parkour, which is very similar to the Step Vault (page 132 onward).

© Michael Schaab

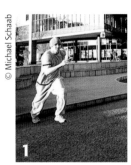
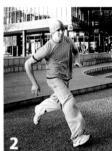
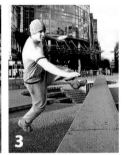
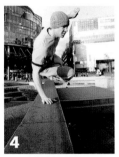
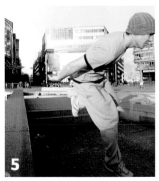
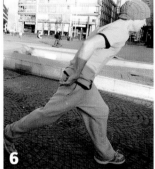
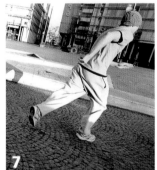

Photo sequence 19: "Basic" Speed (vault)

MOVEMENT DESCRIPTION (SEE PHOTO SEQUENCE 19):

Preparation

1. *Fast approach.*

2. *Right-leg take-off.*

Execution

3. *The left leg is bent as the free leg is pulled up or even kicked out to the side.*

4. *The right hand is supported on the obstacle. The head and upper body are almost parallel to the obstacle during the support phase.*

5. *The right leg (take-off leg) is bent during clearance of the obstacle and then actively pulled to the ground, i.e., the right take-off leg passes the supporting left free leg and touches the ground first.*

Landing

6. *The landing is made in the lunge position so that you can jog away immediately. If the landing is onto a lower level, it is two-footed.*

As mentioned at the start, there is another variation of the Speed that resembles a hurdle clearance technique incorporating a support phase. This technique can also be performed on both sides. We explain this technique with the left support arm and the right take-off leg.

MOVEMENT DESCRIPTION (VARIATION):

Preparation

7. *Fast approach.*

8. *Take off from your right foot far enough away from the obstacle so that the left (free) leg can be brought over the obstacle in front of the body.*

Execution

9. *Use your left hand for support and bend the upper body forward.*

10. *The right take-off leg is brought to the side beside the free leg and is bent over the obstacle.*

Landing

11. *The left leg touches the ground first, the right leg is brought through and touches the ground in front of the left so that you can jog away immediately. If the landing takes place onto a lower level, it is two-footed.*

METHODOLOGY   *A. Outdoors*

Preliminary exercise for the Speed Vault ("Basic"/"hurdle")

- Step Vault

LEARNING STEPS:

1. Running over a knee-high obstacle

Aim: Running take-off and lunge landing so that you can jog away immediately.

Task: Running or jumping over a knee-high obstacle, e.g., a tree stump.

2. Lateral support on a hip-high obstacle with approach

Aim: Lateral support on a hip-high wall/railing with approach.

Task: Acquiring security in the support phase.

3. Step vault over a hip-high wall

4. Speed vault over a hip-high obstacle

Aim: Speed Vault over a hip-high wall.

Task: Demonstration of the target form.

B. Outdoors

Preliminary exercise for the Speed Vault ("Basic"/"hurdle")

- Step Vault

LEARNING STEPS:

1. Running over a knee-high obstacle

Aim: Jumping over an elastic rope or a small box.

Task: Running take-off with lunge landing so that you can jog away immediately.

Apparatus: Lay out flat mats for the landing.

2. Lateral support on a hip-high box with approach

Aim: Lateral support on a hip-high box with approach.

Task: Acquisition of security in the support phase.

Apparatus: *Hip-high* box with mats to the side and rear.

Extension: Tie an elastic rope to the narrow end of the box; the other end is held in a partner's hand.

Task: Approach run, take-off, support on the box and lift your legs to the side to clear the elastic rope.

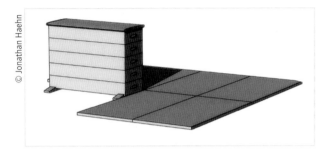

© Jonathan Haehn

3. *Step Vault over a diagonally placed, hip-high box*

4. *Speed Vault over a hip-high obstacle*
Aim: Speed Vault over a diagonally placed, hip-high box.

Task: Demonstration of the target movement.

Apparatus: Diagonally placed, hip-high box with mats behind it.

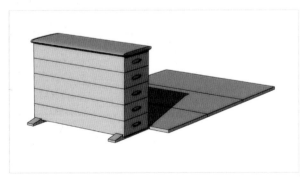

Spotters: A spotter is not usually necessary for these exercises, but it is a good idea to stand behind the box in order to be able to intervene in the case of a fall.

CORRECTING MISTAKES

Observation	Cause	Corrective Actions
Athlete bumps into the box with his legs or hips.	Take-off is not correct.	Faster approach. Higher take-off. The take-off may need to be earlier/farther away from the obstacle.
	Arm does not support the body. Legs/butt too far away from the support hand.	Shoulder should be more above the support hand.
The athlete lands two-footed.	Too little horizontal momentum. Too much vertical momentum.	Faster approach. Low support over the obstacle. Look at the ground as you land and jog away.

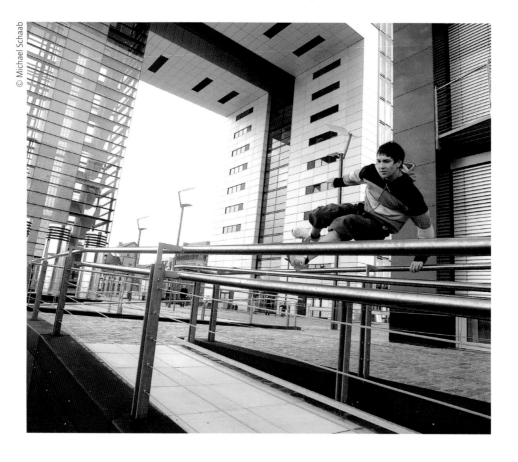

© Michael Schaab

4.5.3   LAZY (VAULT) – PASSEMENT

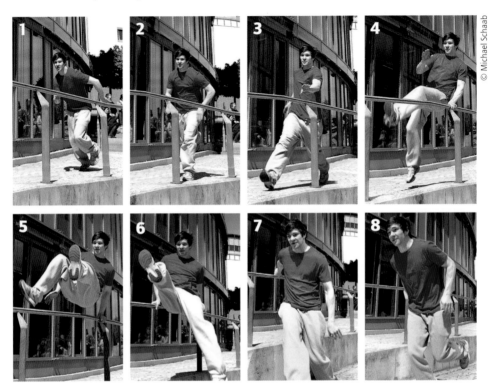

© Michael Schaab

Photo sequence 20: Lazy Vault – passement

MOVEMENT DESCRIPTION:

Preparation

1./2.   Side-on to diagonal approach.

3./4.   One-footed take-off from foot farthest away from the obstacle.

Execution

4./5.   The hand nearest the obstacle is supported on the obstacle, the leg nearest the obstacle swings over it.

6.   Scissor action with the legs with support from the second hand. This introduces the contra body movement, provides stability in the support position and helps the hips to clear the obstacle.

6./7.   The first support hand leaves the obstacle, the second (free) leg prepares for the one-footed landing.

Landing

7./8. Lunge landing so that you can jog away immediately.

TIPS AND TRICKS

- *Lower the center of gravity over the obstacle to avoid losing speed.*
- *Start testing and practicing on narrow walls or railings. Wide walls are slightly harder.*
- *Bring the support arm's shoulder over the support hand in the direction of the movement.*
- *Scissor action with the legs at the center point over the obstacle and swap support hands.*
- *Start off at low speeds and choose lower obstacles. Later, perform from a running start.*

Variations

- "Lazy to Drop" from great heights. Keep the legs together, two-handed directing and push-off in the desired landing direction.

Nothing is impossible

- Lazy Gainer

METHODOLOGY *A. Outdoors*

Preliminary Exercises:

Scissor jump in place. Run over lines and knee-high railings.

LEARNING STEPS:

- Support on hip-high obstacle. Swing up the free leg nearest the obstacle with take-off in front of the obstacle but don't cross it.
- **Extension:** Leg scissors (see above) but from standing position to sitting position on a hip-high wide obstacle (e.g., a wall) with slight body twist in the direction of the movement.
- Whole movement on one level *over* a hip-high, but not too wide wall.

Whole movement on one level over a railing.

Spotter: Usually no help is required for this easy movement. If the athlete wants to cross the obstacle at his first attempt, a helper can stand at the take-off point, hold the first support arm with his hand nearest the obstacle and with the second (helping) hand on the seat/hips, lift and push the body over the obstacle.

B. Indoors

Preliminarv Exercise:

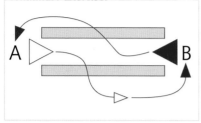

Game of tag on the parallel bars, involving leg scissors over one bar from a diagonal support position, landing and jogging away. Athletes A and B chase each other through the path between the bars across the bars (see diagram).

LEARNING STEPS:

1. *Supported position on two hip-high boxes. Swing up the free leg nearest the obstacle with take-off in front of the obstacle without crossing it.*

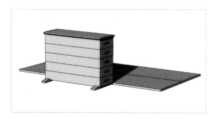

© (2) Jonathan Haehn

Apparatus: Hip-high boxes with mats for safety.

Extension: Support yourself with leg scissors (see above) but then from standing position into sitting position on a hip-high box, slightly twist the body in the direction of movement.

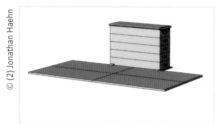

2. *Whole movement on one level over a hip-high box.*

Apparatus: sideways box with mats placed behind it.

3. *Whole movement on one level over a horizontal bar*

Spotter: For this easy movement, no spotter is usually required. If the athlete wants to cross the obstacle at the first attempt, a spotter can stand at the take-off point, hold the first support arm with his hand nearest the obstacle and lift and push the athlete over the obstacle with the other hand on the seat/hips.

Apparatus: Hip-high horizontal bar with mats for safety behind the bar.

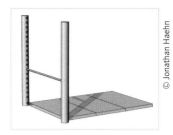

© Jonathan Haehn

Apparatus variations

Support apparatus	Take-off aids
■ bars	■ springboard
■ horse	■ doubled mats
■ balance beam	■ top layer of box

ERROR CORRECTION

Observation	Cause	Corrective Action
Seat touches the obstacle (box).	The second hand does not help to push away from the obstacle.	Think about the change of support hand. The second hand also supports.

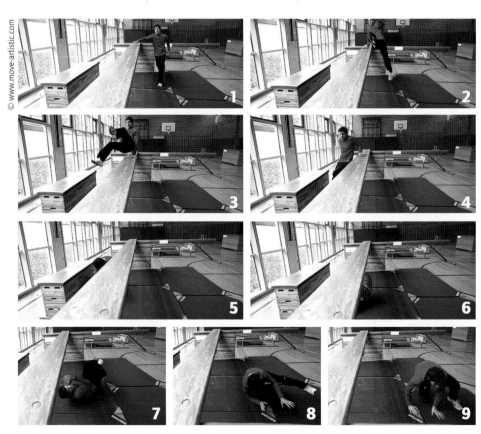

© www.move-artistic.com

Lazy (Vault) followed by roll – example exercise and use of apparatus

4.5.4 KONG (VAULT) "MONKEY" – SAUT DE CHAT

The Kong (Vault) strongly resembles a gymnastics supported tuck jump. But outdoors, there is no springboard and no landing mats. The obstacles and the landing surfaces are hard and allow no room for error.

Neither should you land in a standing position but try to jog away directly. A great deal of courage is required to learn this clearance technique in the outdoors!

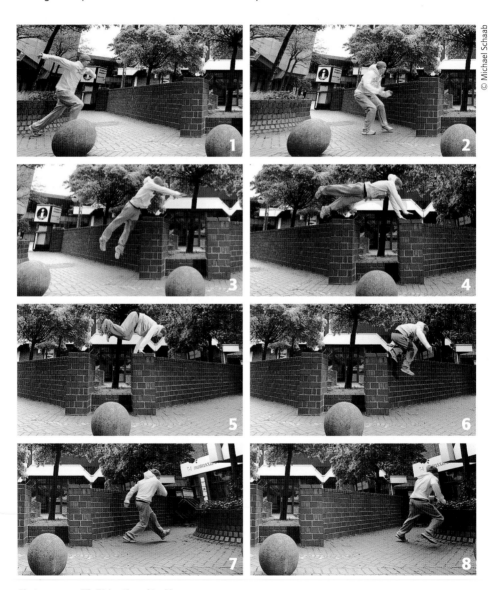

© Michael Schaab

Photo sequence 21: Diving Kong (Vault)

The Kong is very well-suited to clearing wide walls or diving through shoulder-width holes, like windows, when running flat out.

MOVEMENT DESCRIPTION:

Preparation

1. *Approach.*

2. *The take-off can be one-footed, two-footed or from a lunge position. Depending on the take-off technique, the arms are used as swing elements in different ways. The most common take-off technique is probably a lunge take-off with a vigorous arm action. The arms are stretched out in a swinging action toward the obstacle; the upper body is bent slightly forward.*

Execution

3. *First flight phase: arm-torso angle and hip-leg angle are opened and the legs are almost straightened.*

4./5. *Support phase: the hands (attacking-supporting-pulling) are placed in front of the shoulder. The hands may be placed parallel to each other or even one in front of the other. The legs are tucked up toward the chest.*

5./6. *Second flight phase: shoulders and hands push off from the obstacle. This supporting action straightens the upper body up slightly (backward rotation). The feet are brought forward and down, and the eyes focus on the landing spot.*

Landing

7./8. *The landing is either two-footed or in a lunge position so that you can jog away immediately.*

TIPS AND TRICKS

- *In the last third, lean on the support surface.*
- *Bring the hips up in the support phase.*

Variations

- Kong (Vault): take-off surface and support surface at the same height.
- Kong to Precision

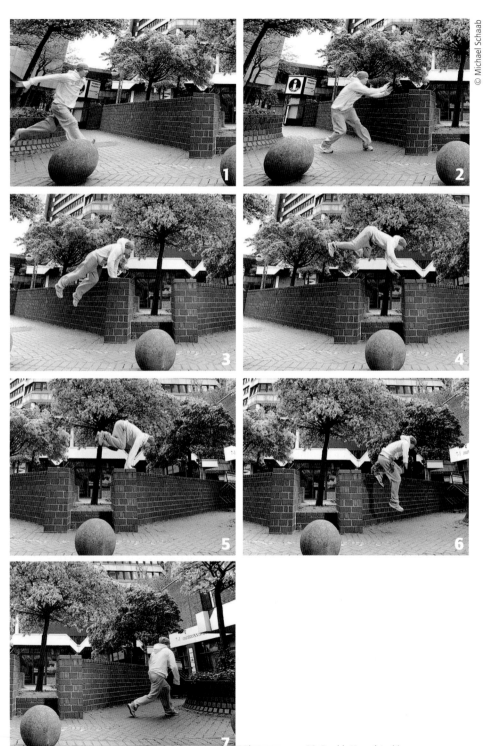

© Michael Schaab

Photo sequence 22: Double Kong (Vault)

- Kong to Cat Leap
- Double Kong

Nothing is impossible

- Triple Kong.
- 360 Kong

METHODOLOGY   *A. Outdoors*

LEARNING STEPS:

1. *Approach, take-off and leg tuck onto a hip-high wall, jump from the wall with controlled landing*
2. *Kong Vault/support tuck jump with spotter over a hip-high wall*

TIP

Push the upper body up high with both hands, keeping your head up!

Spotting position: One or two spotters wait for the athlete behind the wall with outstretched arms. The helpers support the athlete in the sot phase with an upper arm pinch grip (support grip) and pull him over the obstacle if necessary. The spotters support the athlete like this into the standing position, while backing away from the obstacle.

B. Indoors

LEARNING STEPS:

1.   **Tuck jump onto the long box and jump from the box with controlled landing**

Task: The hands rest on a hip-high box, the feet are next to each other. After the tuck jump onto the box, stand up quickly. Take-off from the end of the box into an eccentric, well-controlled landing.

Aim: Practicing the first flight phase and raising the body's center of gravity, prepare for landing.

Apparatus: Place a box longways with mats behind it, then place a box sideways.

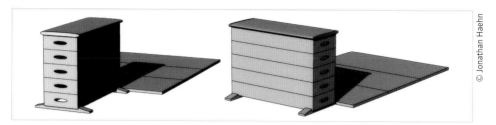

© Jonathan Haehn

Spotting position: Even for this exercise, it can be advisable to use spotters in a manageable and non-dangerous situation. One spotter stands to the left and the other to the right of the longways box. They stretch out their arms toward the approaching athlete in order to quickly take hold of his upper arms in a pinch grip (support grip) (photos 1-3, page 150).

2. Kong (Vault)/saut de chat through an inclined lane

Task: Perform several supports from take-offs through the lane. Simulation of a Kong vault.

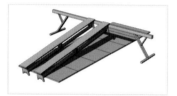

Aim: Support, take-off and raising the center of gravity.

Apparatus: Hang two long benches parallel on a balance beam to create a sloping, shoulder-wide lane. Place mats underneath the lane and behind the beam.

Variation:

In the long bench lane, place obstacles, such as a medicine ball or a small box. Perform a tuck jump over the balance beam with help.

Spotters: One spotter stands to the left and the other to the right behind the beam and they secure the support and dismount with the upper arm pinch grip (see photos 1-3, page 150) to prevent the athlete from falling forward (place small mats behind the beam).

3. Kong (Vault)/saut de chat through a box lane

Task: Take-off (as soon and as far away as possible) in front of the box. The hands rest (as far behind as possible) on both boxes and the athletes tucks his legs up through the box lane.

Aim: Familiarization with heights, take-off and support point (feet cannot be left hanging behind the obstacle).

Apparatus: Two boxes are placed sideways or longways next to each other so that they form a shoulder-width lane.

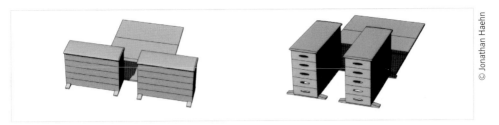

© Jonathan Haehn

Variation:

In the box lane, place obstacles such as a medicine ball or a small box. Later, an elastic rope can also be stretched over the box lane.

Spotters: One helper stands to the right and another to the left alongside the boxes and secures the support and dismount with an upper arm pinch grip (see photos 1-3, page 150), to prevent the athlete from tipping forward (place small mats behind the beam).

4. Approach, Kong over sideways boxes and jog away

Task: Jump over 2-3 sideways boxes in a row as fluidly as possible.

Aim: Kong with and without spotters in the target form.

Apparatus: 2-3 sideways boxes, one behind the other with safety mats behind them (possibly with soft mats to start with).

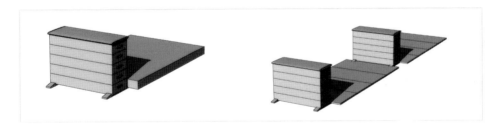

Variation:

Vary the heights of and gaps between two boxes, allowing sufficient room between them. At the end of the vaulting sequence, a roll may be performed.

Spotters: Two spotters wait for the athlete behind the obstacle with their arms outstretched. The helpers support the athlete in the support phase with an upper arm pinch grip (support grip) and pull him over the obstacle if necessary.

The spotter accompanies the athlete into the standing position. The spotters must back away from the obstacle in order to leave the athlete room to land. One spotter may also perform this alone.

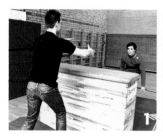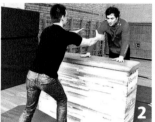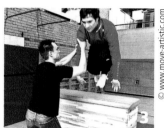

Support grip on the upper arm with both hands

ERROR CORRECTION

Observation	Cause	Corrective Actions
Athlete's feet/seat touch the obstacle.	Hands are placed not far enough back on the obstacle. First flight phase too short.	Mark out the support area with chalk. Try to consciously jump onto the hands in the first flight phase so that you are supported far enough back.
Athlete bangs his knees against the obstacle.	• Take-off not high enough or too near the obstacle. • Possibly not tucking the legs up fast enough.	• Exercise: stand with the hands on the obstacle, then jump up and tuck up the legs.
Backward rotation missing after the support. Athlete falls forward.	• Hands stay on the obstacle for too long. • Too little support strength in the arms. • Too much speed. • Center of gravity is already in front of the shoulders in the support phase.	• Possibly mark out the take-off point. Short, powerful push-off by the hands; don't jump too high into the support phase.
Cannot jog away after landing, athlete lands on both feet.	Backward lean on landing due to body straightening too soon.	Lean the upper body farther forward on landing. Look forward and down at the ground.

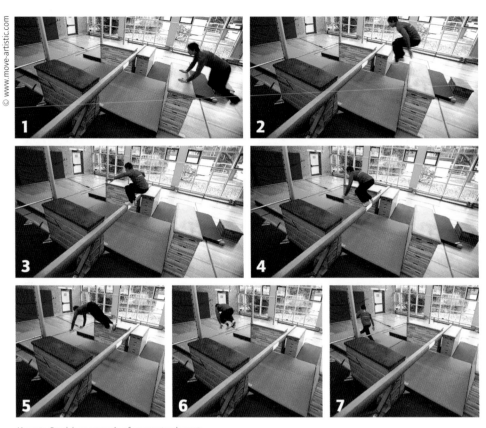

Kong to Precision: example of apparatus layout

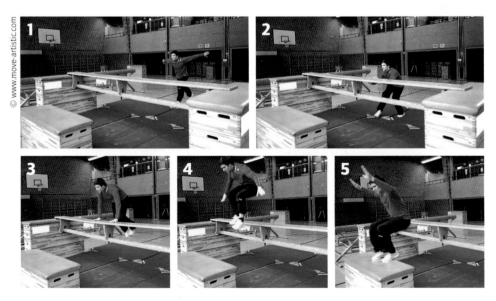

Kong to Precision – alternative apparatus layout

4.5.5   DASH (VAULT) – PASSEMENT ASSIS

The Dash (Vault) is a combination of jumping and supporting techniques and is very similar to the Lazy (Vault). First, the athlete tries to clear the obstacle from a head-on approach and a leap, while the hips and leg are brought forward, with a support added just before the end of the clearance.

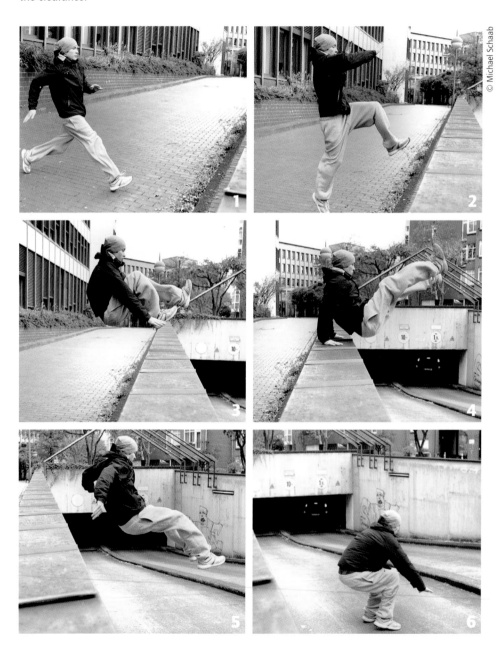

© Michael Schaab

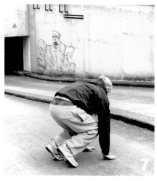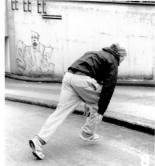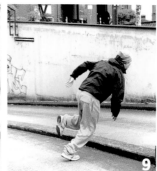

Photo sequence 23: Dash (Vault)

MOVEMENT DESCRIPTION:

Preparation

1.   Approach.

2.   The one-foot take-off must be performed far enough before the obstacle so that the legs have room to be tucked up in front of it because the legs cross the obstacle first. The upper body leans slightly back at take-off, the belly button moves skyward.

Execution

3.   The upper body is upright as it clears the obstacle and the legs are tucked up.

4.   The hands support below and just behind the hips with straight arms.

4./5.   Pushing off the obstacle supports the forward motion.

5.   The legs are straightened toward the ground in the second flight phase.

Landing

6.-9.   If the second flight phase is downward, you can also land on two feet (photos 6-9). In a landing in the lunge position, one leg is actively placed on the ground in order to go into a lunge position and jog away after the support.

TIPS AND TRICKS

■ Jump as flat as possible over the obstacle to minimize loading on the supporting arms (wrists, elbows and shoulder joints).

Nothing is impossible

■ Dash Bomb

METHODOLOGY   *A. Outdoors*

Preliminary Exercise:

Lazy Vault over a hip-high wall with side-on to diagonal approach.

Note: (valid for outdoors and indoors): Lazy and Dash are fundamentally similar techniques. The key differences are the approach angle and speed. If you master the Lazy with a *diagonal* approach to the obstacle, one way of gradually trying out the Dash is by increasing the approach angle every time you perform the exercise until your approach is finally head-on.

LEARNING STEPS:

1. *From a head-on approach, jump over a low obstacle.*
2. *Sit on the wall and then push off into a lunge position so that you can jog away immediately.*
3. *Jump over the wall supporting yourself from behind, two-footed landing then jog.*
4. *Dash (Vault) technique, one-footed landing into lunge position.*

B. Indoors

LEARNING STEPS:

1. *Jumping over a low obstacle with head-on approach*
Apparatus: Lay out small boxes with sufficient distance between them.

2. *Spotters lift the athlete over a hip-high obstacle*
Aim: To get a feel for the movement sequence, particularly the early take-off and to bring the hips forward.

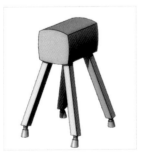

Apparatus: Hip-high vaulting buck. No mats are usually necessary. Spotters may trip over the edges of the mats.

Spotters: Two spotters take the athlete's hand and upper arm and run with him. When he takes off and brings his legs forward, the spotters carry him over the buck.

Verbal encouragement:

■ *"tummy towards the ceiling!"*

■ *"active landing one foot after the other!"*

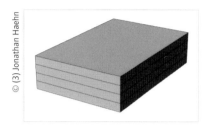

© (3) Jonathan Haehn

3. Approach; one-foot jump onto a "mat pile" in a sitting position with the legs out straight

Apparatus: Mat pile 3-4 thick mats placed on top of each other or two thick mats on three parallel gym benches.

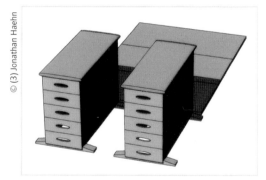

© (3) Jonathan Haehn

4.   Dash through a box lane

Apparatus: shoulder-width box lane with two hip-high boxes placed longways. Mats on the floor behind the box lane.

Extension by placing obstacles in the box lane. First jump over a small box, then support on the boxes.

5. Jump over an elastic rope stretched across the box lane

Apparatus: See step 5 with an elastic rope stretched in the middle of the box lane.

Spotter: Move with the athlete with the upper arm pinch grip beside the box lane if necessary (the spotter takes a lot of momentum out of the movement and is often found to get in the way).

Alternative: The spotter can also first intervene in the support phase to stop the athlete from falling backward.

6. Jumping over the obstacle with the Dash (Vault) technique, landing on the run

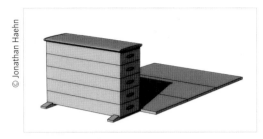

© Jonathan Haehn

Apparatus: Sideways hip-high box with mats placed behind it.

Spotter: Support the athlete on take-off at the hips and back to facilitate the jump over the obstacle and bring the hips forward. The spotter(s) stands at the take-off point, grips the upper arm with the hand nearest the box and the far hand under the seat/ hips pushes the center of gravity over the box.

ERROR CORRECTION

Observation	Cause	Corrective Actions
Athlete's legs hang over the obstacle.	Take-off too close to the obstacle, the legs can no longer be brought over the obstacle.	Take off farther away from the obstacle (possibly mark take-off point on the floor).
The athlete does not adopt the support position.	The athlete jumps too high over the obstacle.	Jump as flat as possible over the obstacle, lean the upper body slightly backward and point your belly button up.

4.5.6   KASH (VAULT)

The Kash is a combination of a **K**ong and a **D**ash. The Kash is used to clear roughly **hip to shoulder height and width obstacles**. If it is no longer possible to clear an obstacle with a Kong or a Dash due to its height, then it may still be possible with a Kash as it is performed with a second supporting movement.

The aim of the first support phase (photos 4/5) is to bring the center of gravity above the support point so that the legs can be tucked up before the second support point. It works better if the hands are lifted off the obstacle after the first support to give the legs more space (double support). The aim of the second support phase is to keep the hips above the support point and push them forward after the support as in a Dash (photos 6/7).

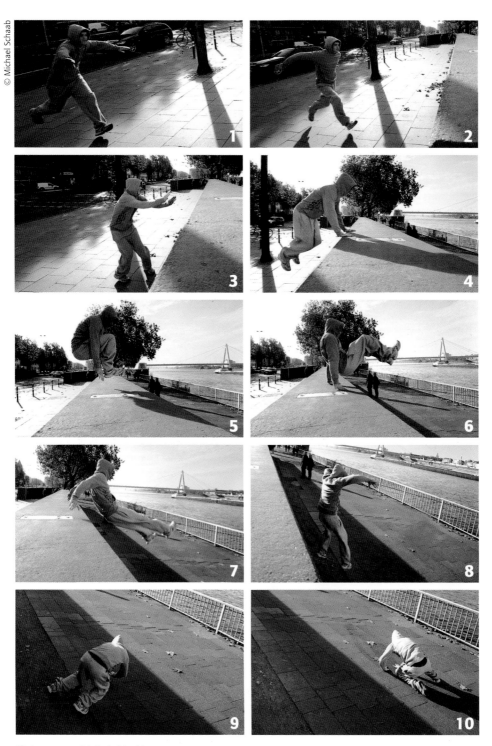

© Michael Schaab

Photo sequence 24: Kash (Vault)

MOVEMENT DESCRIPTION:

Preparation

1. *Head-on approach to the obstacle.*
2. *Take-off from two feet or lunge position. The arms swing back parallel to gain momentum.*
3. *The foot/feet take(s) off relatively close to the obstacle, the arms are now in front of the body.*

Execution

4. *The hands are shoulder-width apart for the support phase.*
5. *Energetic push-off from the shoulders and with the hands from the obstacle, then the legs are tucked up close to the stomach and the feet are brought forward over the obstacle.*
6. *Second support.*
7. *Second push off the obstacle and stretching forward of the body/legs for landing.*

Landing

8./10. *The landing is adapted to the height and the landing surface.*

METHODOLOGY   *A. Outdoors*

Prerequisites/Preliminary Exercises:

■ Kong Vault
■ Dash Vault

LEARNING STEPS:

Outdoors, it is advisable to approach this movement very carefully.

1. *From a head-on approach, tuck up onto a narrow, hip-high wall.*
2. *From a head-on approach, tuck jump over a narrow, hip-high wall.*
3. *In the Kash movement, try out a Kong (page 144) in the first support and a Speed exit (page 134) after the second support.*
4. *Tuck jump over a wall with double support and push off from the wall.*
5. *Approach, see step 4, but push off higher from the first support in order to bring the legs forward sooner in a tuck position under the body.*
6. *Kash over a hip to chest-high wall.*

7. *See step 6, but choose a wider wall.*

8. *See steps 6 and 7, but vary the landing depth.*

B. Outdoors

LEARNING STEPS:

1. *Kong over a sideways box (page 144 onward)*

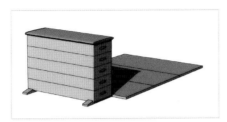

Apparatus: sideways, hip-high box with mats behind it.

2. *Dash over a sideways box (page 152 onward)*

Apparatus: See step 1.

3. *Kash in box lane*

Apparatus: Shoulder-width box lane with two longways, hip-high boxes. Place mats behind the boxes.

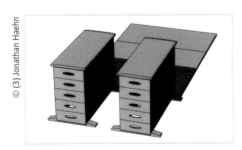

Extension by placing obstacles in the box lane: Kash over small obstacles in box lane.

4. *Kong over sideways box into sitting position with straight legs on mat pile*

Apparatus: Pile of 3-4 soft mats directly behind a sideways hip-high box.

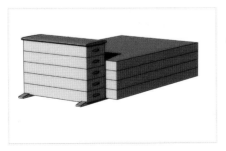

5. *See step 4 with two support phases on the box*

Apparatus: See under 4.

© (3) Jonathan Haehn

6. *Kong with double support, where the legs are brought forward between the support movements. Land on the box in the sitting position (Tip: keep your approach short)*

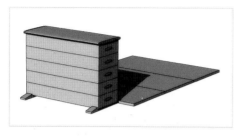

Apparatus: Sideways, hip-high box with small mats behind it.

7. *Kash over a sideways box*

Apparatus: See step 6.

8. *Kash over "box table"*

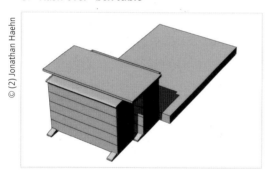

© (2) Jonathan Haehn

Apparatus: Two boxes placed side by side with a firm small mat placed on top.

No spotter: A spotter is not really needed for this movement as a support grip is restricting and usually blocks the movement instead of helping it.

ERROR CORRECTION

Observation	Cause	Corrective Actions
Athlete's feet hang for too long over the box.	Too little push off from the box in the first support phase so that the legs cannot be tucked up and brought through.	Push upwards rather than forward away from the box.
Athlete's seat hangs for too long over the obstacle.	Athlete collapses on the second support and cannot support his bodyweight.	Push the hips forward over the obstacle in the second support phase.

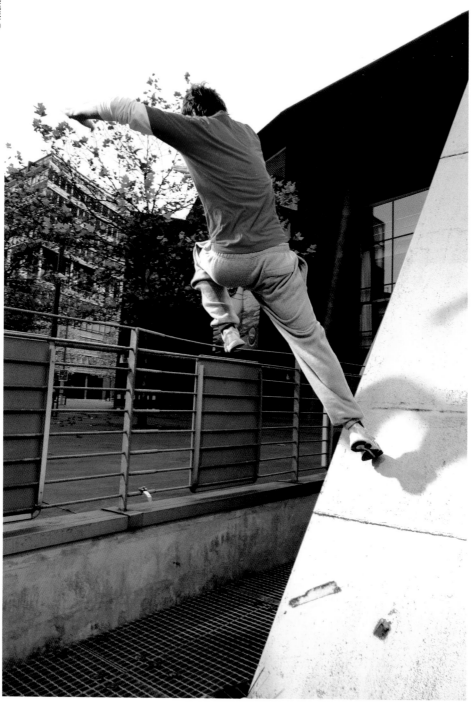

4.5.7   REVERSE (VAULT) – PASSEMENT ARRIÈRE

The Reverse is a support jump from a head-on approach followed by a rotation around the longitudinal axis and a landing with the back to the obstacle before jogging away. It is particularly suited to short approaches or as a final move, e.g., after a preceding Kong over a second obstacle. This technique is also a good way of introducing a change of direction on or after the landing.

There are different ways of performing this support technique. As with most support techniques, the take-off technique can also be varied in the Reverse. The turning direction around the body's longitudinal axis can also be varied. In addition, support can either be provided by one or two hands. The landing strategy must be adapted to the conditions.

However, a basic technique does exist, which is described in the paragraphs below.

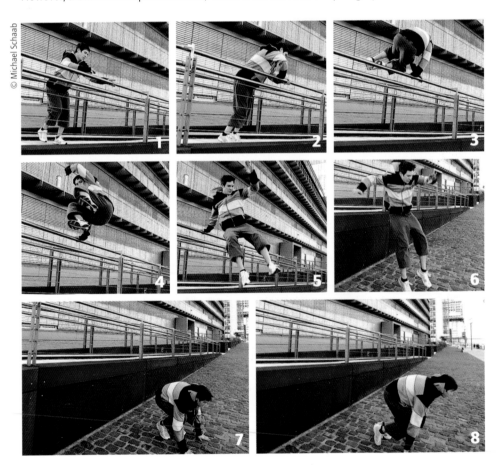

© Michael Schaab

Photo sequence 25: Reverse

MOVEMENT DESCRIPTION:

Preparation

1. Take-off from one foot, two feet or lunge position.
2. Body rotation starts at take-off: the arms and upper body are turned in the direction of rotation.

Execution

2./3. The hands are placed next to each other or one in front of the other, and the (front) support hand pushes off second and is turned in the direction of rotation. In the support position, the front shoulder moves over the rotated support hand. The first support hand is raised very early from the obstacle.

4./5. In the support phase, it is the head that controls the rotation. The rear hand supports the rotation by pushing off. The upper body turns so the back is facing the obstacle. The body remains compact during rotation; the knees are pulled toward the chest.

5. The preparation for landing is supported by a gentle push from the obstacle by the turned support hand.

6. The body opens out during the rotation around the longitudinal axis so that the back is facing the obstacle and stretches out to prepare for landing.

Landing

7./8. The landing strategy is dependent upon the depth of the landing area. If it is on the same level, the landing can be two-footed or in the lunge position. If there is a height difference, the landing can also be followed by a PK roll.

TIPS AND TRICKS

- The movement is controlled by the head and the looking direction: turn your head quickly toward the landing area.
- Your free arm, which was first to be put down and then lifted up, supports the rotation.
- Stay compact during the rotation! Pull your knees into your chest.
- Push yourself actively off the obstacle with the turned hand.
- A Reverse over a wall is easier than a Reverse over a railing.

Variations

- One-handed Reverse

- Tuck jump onto a long obstacle and Reverse dismount (combination of tuck jump and Reverse)
- Reverse with complete longitudinal rotation after support

Nothing is impossible
Reverse followed by landing in Cat-Leap position.

METHODOLOGY *A. Outdoors*

Pre requisite:
Reverse on/over with hands placed one behind the other followed by landing.

LEARNING STEPS:
1. *Approach, place the hands one behind the other for support and Reverse Vault onto the wall.*
2. *Approach, take-off and tuck the legs up to the side onto a narrow, hip-high wall. The rear, first-placed support hand is lifted from the wall, dismount with rotation around the longitudinal axis and land with your back to the wall.*
3. *Reverse sideways with the body/legs over a hip-high wall.*
4. *Reverse over a wall with spotter.*

Spotter: The spotter waits for the athlete behind the wall and secures the landing by holding the hips with a pinch grip (see Indoors).

5. *Reverse without spotter with different landing techniques.*

B. Indoors

LEARNING STEPS:
1. *Approach, support with hands one behind the other and tuck jump onto the box*
Apparatus: Sideways, hip high box with small mats placed behind it for safety.

2. *Approach, take-off and sideways tuck onto a sideways, hip-high box. Lift the rear,*

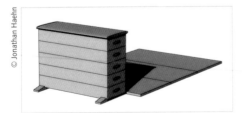

first-placed support hand from the box; tuck the legs during the rotation around the longitudinal axis and land with your back to the box.
Apparatus: See under 1.

© Jonathan Haehn

3. *Approach, hands placed one behind the other for support, Reverse sideways with the body/legs over a box (support over the narrow end of box)*

Apparatus: Sideways, hip-high box with mats placed to the side and rear.

4. *Approach, take-off, Reverse in a wide box lane with elastic rope*

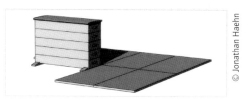

© Jonathan Haehn

Apparatus: Box lane with two hip-high boxes. Place an elastic rope (e.g., rope, rubber band) across the center of the box lane. Place small mats for safety in and behind the wide box lane.

5. *Approach, take-off, Reverse over the box with take-off aid (e.g., trampette, springboard or box top) and spotter*

Apparatus: Sideways, hip-high box with small mats or a large built-in spring mat behind the box for safety. Plac a take-off aid in front of the box if required.

Spotter: The spotter waits for the athlete behind the box and supports the last phase of the rotation and secures the landing with a pinch grip on the hips.

© www.move-artistic.com

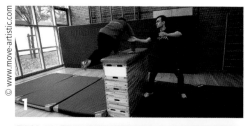

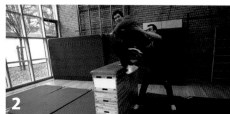

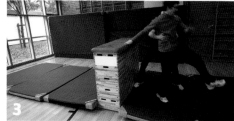

6. Reduce take-off aids and spotting

Apparatus: Sideways hip-high box with mats placed behind it for safety.

© Jonathan Haehn

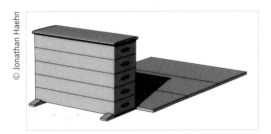

ERROR CORRECTION

Observation	Cause	Corrective Actions
The athlete crosses the obstacle looking to the side, which often pulls him to the side or makes him fall to the side when landing.	• Incomplete rotation. • Lack of control during landing.	• The looking direction controls the movement. Look in the desired movement direction as soon as possible. • Pull the free arm decisively in the direction of movement.

4.5.8   TURN (VAULT) – DEMI-TOUR

It is not easy to generalize about the technique of the Turn Vault (demi-tour) because there are a few variations of the technique. However, it involves a supported rotation, usually over a hip-high railing, then a hang from the railing and a drop to a lower level.

General advice:

- The take-off can be one or two-footed.
- One can twist to the left or to the right.
- The supported rotation is mainly around one arm, while the other hand moves.
- The feet can land simultaneously or one after the other.

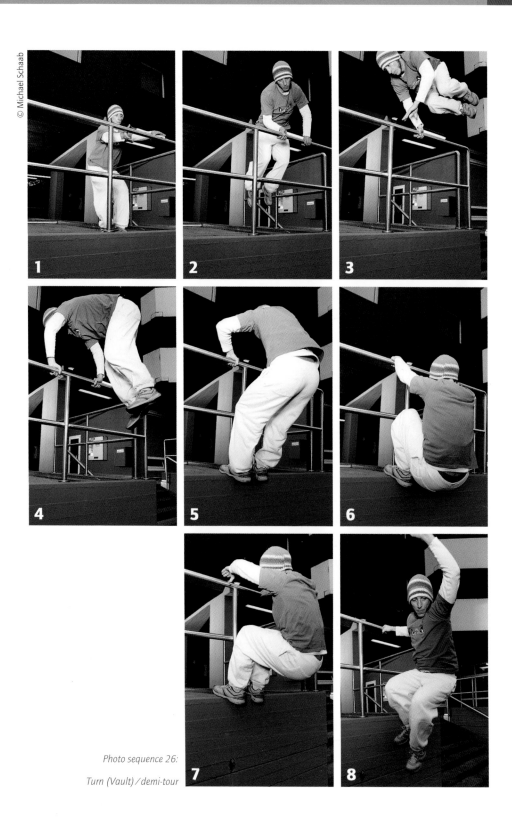

© Michael Schaab

Photo sequence 26:

Turn (Vault)/demi-tour

MOVEMENT DESCRIPTION:

Preparation

1. *Grip the railing with both hands, with the support hand/turning arm twisted around (mixed grip): if you turn to the left, then support yourself on your left arm; if you turn to the right, support with your right arm. With the other hand, pull on the railing in order to gain some momentum and to pull your upper body in the direction of rotation. The pull of the arms and the take-off with the legs must be almost simultaneous in order to get the hips over the railing.*

2. *Take-off with extension of the twisted support arm and push-off from the non-twisting arm to support the twisting push-off*

Execution

3. *In the support phase, change your grip/move your hand and turn around the support arm over the railing. In the support point, the legs are tucked up over the pole or in the scissors position (you can also scissor/roll both legs one after the other over the pole). For a moment, all the bodyweight is supported by the support arm. The push-off arm moves in the one-armed support phase, when speed is of the essence.*

4. *With the grip of the outside hand changing, the upper body is turned through up to 180° in order to prepare early for the landing, during which it is advisable to carefully lower the center of gravity from the support after the hand change*

5. *The feet quickly (already during the twisting action) look for a grip on the wall (at the bottom of the railing). The feet can either be placed side by side simultaneously or one after the other (also one on top of the other).*

Landing

5./6. *If you have a good grip on the railing and a firm grip with the feet, the center of gravity can also be lowered into the knee hang position (Cat-Leap – photo 6).*

Tip: If the movement is perfected and you are going to try it out in familiar terrain, then don't lower your center of gravity slowly but jump directly into the knee hang position.

WATCH OUT!

This should only be done on very stable terrain because the pulling forces are very high and there is a risk of uprooting the railing.

7./8. *From this position, jump with another 180° turn down to the lower level (dismount/ saut de fond). Concentration and control are key for the landing!*

METHODOLOGY **A. Outdoor**

LEARNING STEPS:

First, find a narrow wall or railing on a level

1. *From a standing start, take-off, push yourself over a railing (with the left arm, right arm and with both arms).*
2. *From a running start, take-off and push yourself over a railing with a 180° turn.*
3. *From a standing start with a 180° turn and changing hand grip, push yourself over the railing.*
4. *Turn (Vault)/demi-tour on a railing to knee hang followed by drop/dismount (page 167).*
5. *Experiment with these variations:*
    - one-foot take-off
    - two-foot take-off
    - two-foot landing on the other side of the railing
    - one foot lands after the other on the other side of the railing
    - for advanced practitioners: turn around your weaker side

Spotter: A spotter may assist the athlete at the support phase. The spotter stands at the take-off point and grips the support arm around the upper arm below the shoulder. The leg tuck can be supported by a push on the back of the thigh of the leg nearest the body (see Indoors).

B. Outdoor

LEARNING STEPS:

Apparatus layout: For the learning steps below, you can use hip-high horizontal bars, a single bar from a set of parallel bars (remove the second one) and a balance beam. The landing area should be covered with mats.

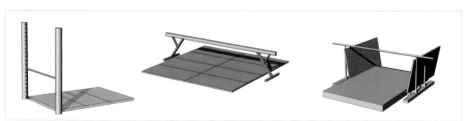

© Jonathan Haehn

1. *Running start, take-off and support/push over with the right hand.*

2. *Running start, take-off and support/push over with the left hand.*

3. *Standing take-off. Support over the horizontal bar or the balance beam (with the left, right and/or both hands).*

4. *Running start, support over horizontal bar or balance beam with a 180° turn.*

5. *Standing start, support over horizontal bar or balance beam with a 180° turn (without exact technical instructions).*

6. *Introduction of the Turn (Vault)/demi-tour – explanation of the hand position. Demonstrate movement and show variations if possible.*

7. *Try out these variations:*

   - one-footed take-off
   - two-footed take-off
   - two-footed landing
   - land one foot after the other and
   - for advanced practitioners: rotate around the other (weaker) side

Spotter: The athlete can be supported by a spotter who grips the support arm around the upper arm below the shoulder. The leg tuck can be supported by a push on the hips or back of the thigh of the leg nearest the spotter.

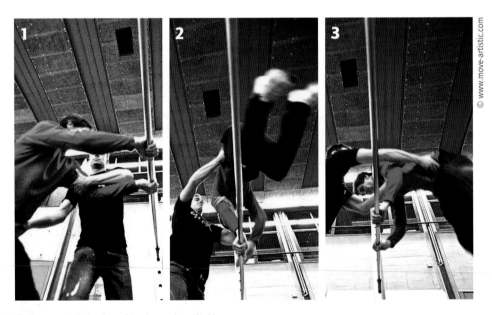

© www.move-artistic.com

Half over arm pinch grip and turning push on the hips.

ERROR CORRECTION

Observation	Cause	Corrective Action
The athlete's feet or shins remain hanging on the bar.	This can have many causes: • Inadequate jumping power or supporting strength • The center of gravity is too far away from the support/pivot arm • Simple fear of falling	• Make the movement easier by using a take-off aid (e. g., springboard) • Help from a spotter in the support phase. • Bring the shoulders farther over the support hand.

© www.move-artistic.com

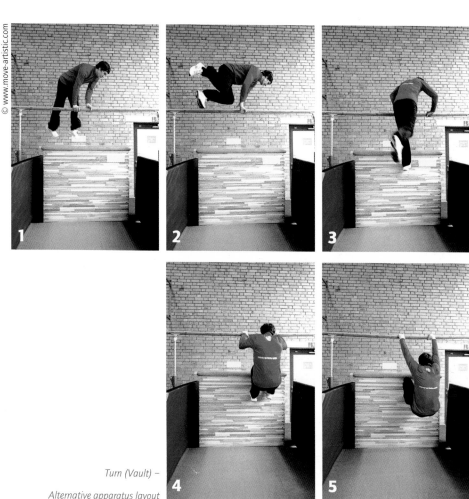

Turn (Vault) –
Alternative apparatus layout

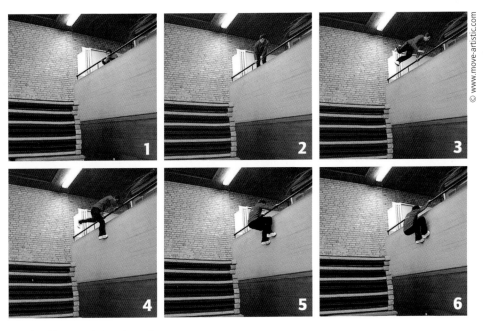

Turn (Vault) – example for advanced traceurs

4.5.9   PALM SPIN

The Palm Spin resembles a crouched, rotating dismount in gymnastics. This movement is not an efficient vaulting technique and can therefore be considered more of a Freerunning move.

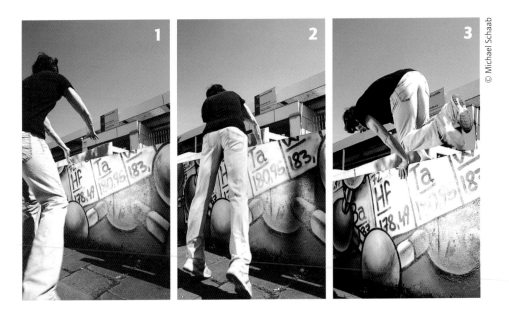

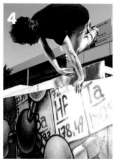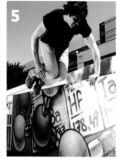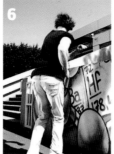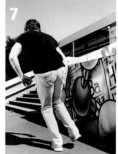

Photo sequence 27: Palm Spin

MOVEMENT DESCRIPTION:

Preparation

1. *Head-on or slightly angled approach to the obstacle.*
2. *Two-footed take-off (most frequent variation).*

Execution

3./5. *Two-handed support using mixed grip, pivot hand turned out (or one-handed support with the fingers of the pivot hand pointing in the direction of movement or in a turned overhand grip in the case of a railing). With the take off, the other hand gives a push in the direction of movement and is brought into the body as a rotation support. Turn around the support arm with the legs tucked up close to the abdomen.*

Landing

5./7. *Body extension to prepare for landing, which may be one-footed or two-footed facing the obstacle.*

TIPS AND TRICKS

■ *Guide the hips up over the support area of the hand.*

■ *Look at the support hand during take-off and at the ground during the supported rotation.*

■ *The shoulder should stay in front of the support hand.*

■ *The second hand initiates the rotation and is pulled into the body during the support phase to support the turning movement.*

■ *Look for a take-off point that is higher than the landing area.*

■ *Head-on approach.*

Variations

- Palm spin on a railing.
- Palm spin to change direction (with your back to the obstacle).
- Palm spin as 360° turn landing with your back to the obstacle in order to reengage with the obstacle.

A. Outdoors

Preliminary Exercises

- Turn/demi-tour over a wall.

LEARNING STEPS:

1. *Two-footed take-off from a standing start or a short approach run. Tuck jump over a wall corner: take-off from the short side or the long side of the wall, depending on the conditions. Both hands grip the edge of a wall, the thumbs of both hands point toward the wall edge. Take-off, side vault with almost a half turn onto the wall. Tuck jump with turn over the corner of the wall. The upper body undergoes a 270° rotation in this drill.*
2. *From a short approach, two-foot take-off, Palm spin over the corner of a wall. Hands grip the edge of the wall, as in the first learning step (if necessary, with a spotter).*

Spotter: Half upper arm pinch grip, push/turn the hips to aid rotation (see photos 1 and 2, page 175).

3. *Approach, two-foot take-off, Palm spin on the short side of the wall (if necessary, with a spotter). Support with a two-handed mixed grip, pivot hand turned out. The other hand gives a push in the direction of movement and is brought into the body to support rotation.*

Spotter: Half upper arm pinch grip, turn push the hips to aid rotation (see photos 1 and 2, page 175).

4. *Approach, take-off, Palm spin on the long side of the wall (if necessary, with a spotter).*
5. *Approach, take-off, Palm spin on a hip-high railing (if necessary, with a spotter).*

B. Indoors

Preliminary Exercises

■ Turn/demi-tour over a horse.

Apparatus: The learning steps are performed over a hip-high box. Mats should be placed on the landing area.

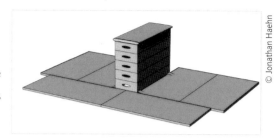

© Jonathan Haehn

LEARNING STEPS:

1. *From a standing start or a short approach, two-footed take-off, tuck jump over one corner of the box: take-off in front of the short side of the box. Both hands grip one corner of the box, the thumbs of both hands point toward the box corner. Take-off, turn with almost half turn onto the box. Leg tuck and rotation from box. The upper body undergoes a 270° turn with this drill.*

2. *From a short approach, two-foot take-off, Palm spin over a corner of the box (first with and then without take-off aid, e.g., springboard). Hands grip the corner of the box.*

Spotter: Half upper arm pinch grip and turn/push the hips to aid rotation.

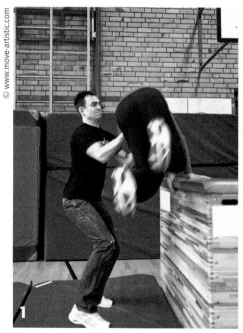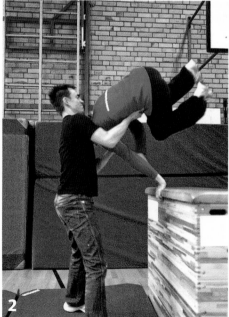

© www.move-artistic.com

Half upper arm pinch grip and pushing/turning the hips.

3. *Approach run, two-footed take-off, Palm spin on the short side of the box with spotter and take-off aid. Two-handed, mixed grip support, pivot hand turned out. Other hand gives a push in the direction of movement and is brought close to the body to support rotation.*

Spotter: Half upper arm pinch grip, turn and push the hips to aid rotation.

4. *Approach, take-off, Palm spin without spotter and take-off aid on the short side of the box.*
5. *Approach, take-off, Palm spin on the long side of the box (if necessary, with a spotter).*
6. *Approach, take-off, Palm spin on a hip-high horizontal bar (if necessary, with a spotter).*

ERROR CORRECTION

Observation	Cause	Corrective Action
The athlete's legs hang on the box during the supported rotation.	• The hips are not high enough above the obstacle during the supported rotation.	• Concentrate on a high take-off. Keep your hips high and look down.
	• The shoulders are above (instead of in front of) the obstacle, thus shifting the center of gravity too far over the obstacle.	• Keep the shoulders in front of the obstacle by pushing away from the obstacle with the support arms.

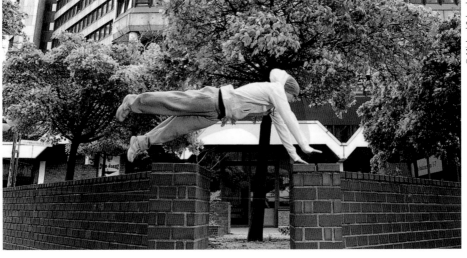

© Michael Schaab

4.6 CLIMBING – GRIMPER

Climbing, along with running, racing, jumping and landing, is one of the most important basic skills in Parkour and should therefore be trained in a variety of ways.

Climbing without security should always be learned and practiced at ground level. Falls when climbing can have serious consequences, hence the basic rule, "don't climb up higher than you can jump down!"

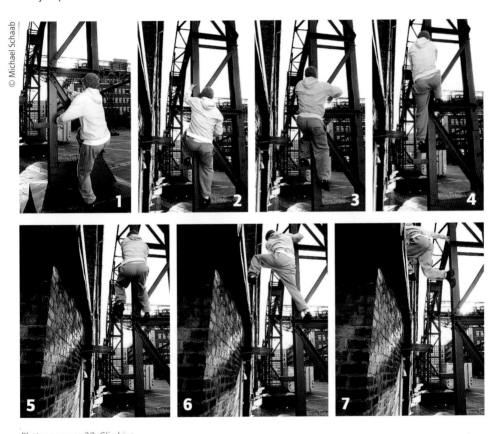

Photo sequence 28: Climbing

In this chapter we shall only describe Parkour-specific climbing, not basic climbing techniques. The authors have listed all Parkour climbing techniques in which the emphasis is on climbing up combined with climbing on top of things, or climbing as almost vertical movement.

This chapter contains more detailed descriptions of the Wall Run, Cat Leap/Arm Jump, Muscle-Up and Wall Dismount.

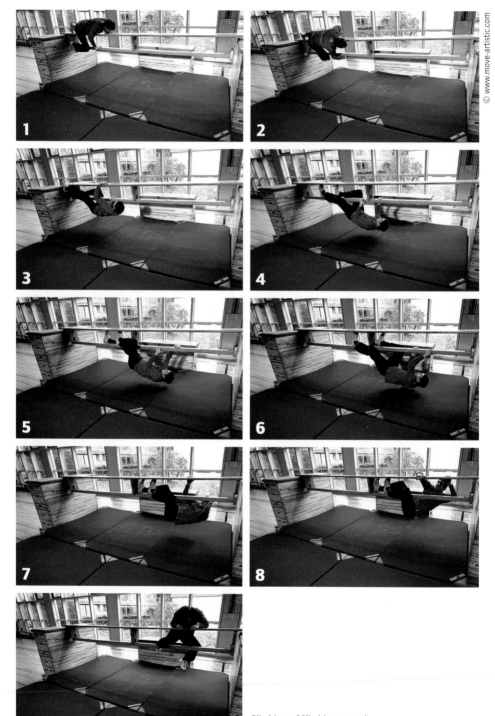

© www.move-artistic.com

Climbing – "Climbing around a gym bench" an example exercise in the gym.

4.6.1 WALL RUN/WALL-UP – PASSE MURAILLE

The Wall Run is a technique that is used to **climb or clear walls as fast as possible**. It is a very efficient technique that requires a fast, powerful push off and up the wall and enough strength in the arms, shoulders and upper body to be able to push up into an arm support on top of the wall at the end of the movement. The Wall Run is a complex movement combination consisting of an approach, take-off, climb, gripping/hanging and push up to support.

© Michael Schaab

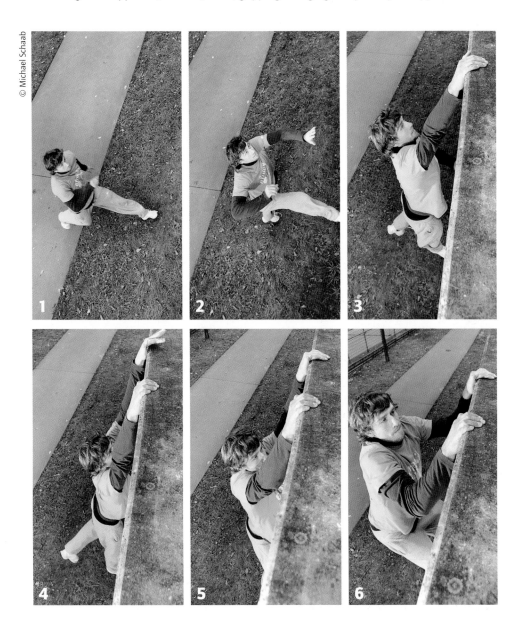

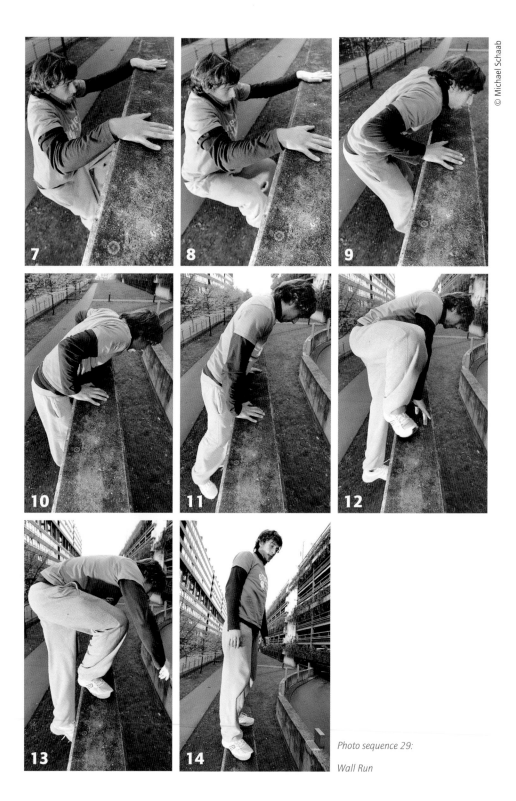

© Michael Schaab

Photo sequence 29:

Wall Run

MOVEMENT DESCRIPTION:

Preparation

1.   Approach. One-footed take-off in front of the wall about one leg length away in order to be able to divert the horizontal momentum with the step/stride onto the wall efficiently into a vertical direction with no loss of speed.

Execution

2.   The ball of the foot of the free leg is placed against the wall, the body is upright and relatively close to the wall. The free leg now becomes the push-off leg that straightens to push the body upward.

3./4. If possible, both arms grip the top of the obstacle. Alternatively, grip the top of the obstacle with one hand, so that you can reach a greater height due to the diagonal stretch. The second hand should follow the first as quickly as possible.

5.-7. In the hanging position, the balls of the feet are placed against the wall and they push quickly off the wall to support the pull-up movement of the arms.

6.-10. As soon as your chest is level with the top of the wall, you should move your hands and place them flat on the top of it. Next bring your chest over your hands to make it easier to push yourself up into the support position.

Landing

11./12. In the support position, place one foot to the side of your hand on the wall.

13.   Straighten the leg on the wall, and stand upright while pulling your second leg up.

14.   The movement is completed when you are standing still on top of the wall.

TIPS AND TRICKS

If you are not strong enough for this technique, you can also bring one elbow over the edge of the wall and pull the second one after it then push yourself up into the support position from there.

Variations

■ Wall Hop: Approach, one-footed take-off in front of the wall. Step/stride onto the side of the wall to gain height. Lean on the hands with direct tuck jump onto or over a chest to head-height wall.

© Michael Schaab

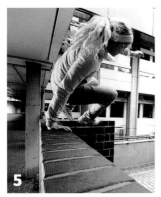
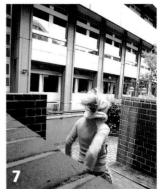
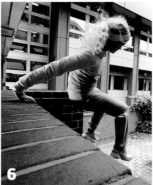
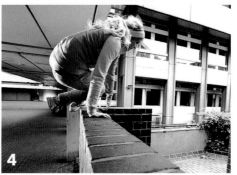
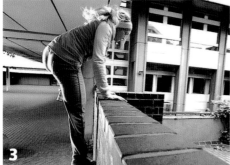
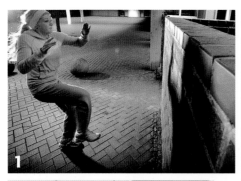
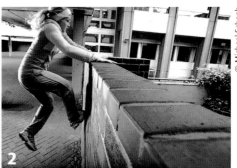

Photo sequence 30: Wall Hop

Nothing is impossible

360° Wall Up (step onto a wall with 360° rotation around the longitudinal axis then grip the edge of the wall).

METHODOLOGY *A. Outdoors*

LEARNING STEPS:

1. *From a 3-5 stride approach, take off with your "weak" take-off leg roughly one leg-length away from the wall and step onto the wall with your "strong" take-off leg.*

   Aim: Learn to gain height.

   Tips: Land on the wall with the balls of your feet. Do not push away from the wall.

   Variation/consolidation: Two steps against the wall with 180° turn, landing and roll back to the starting point.

2. *From a short approach run, step up onto the wall in order to gain height. Grip the top edge of the wall with your hands. Push yourself up into the support position. You can make this movement easier by taking specific steps up the wall.*

   Tip: If the wall height is optimal (to suit the height and ability of the athlete), the step onto the wall can be supported by *simultaneously gripping* the top edge and the *free leg action*, so that the hips easily clear the top of the wall. It is then easy to tuck jump on top or even over the wall.

   Advice: The safe performance of a wall dismount is a necessary skill that should also be practiced as a follow-up exercise (page 194 onward).

   Of course, it is also possible to perform a drop with PK roll.

B. Indoors

LEARNING STEPS:

The wall run cannot be practiced correctly in every gym, because of the lack of appropriate walls or edges to grip, let alone a big enough ledge 2-3 yards high on which to support oneself. The following two methodological steps can almost always be practiced as preliminary exercises for a wall run (make sure that enough mats are placed in front of the wall).

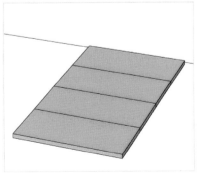

© Jonathan Haehn

1. *From a 3-5 stride approach, take-off from your "weak" take-off leg roughly one leg-length from the wall and step onto the wall with your "strong" take-off leg.*

   Aim: Learn to gain height.

   Tips: Land on the wall with the balls of your feet. Don't push away from the wall.

   Variation/Consolidation: Two steps against the wall with 180° rotation, land and roll back to the starting position.

2. *The hands grip as high up as possible.*

Alternative Methodology

Some gyms have seating that may be used. Some have enough (stiff) mats, such as judo mats, with which a *mat pile* can be built on which you can practice the Wall Run into support position (see Outdoors methodology) then climb on top. Alternatively, the foundation of a mat pile can be formed with three boxes to make it easier to build. The disadvantage of a box foundation is that the wooden surface is relatively slippery and offers little friction for

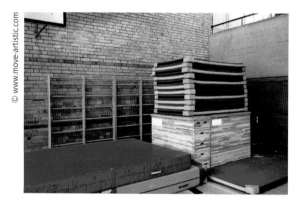

the purposes of pushing off. However, this structure provides the desired effect of testing and training upper body strength. It is also important that the mats, whether judo mats or small mats, have a relatively firm top edge.

Mat piles should be surrounded by mats for safety.

Example of a mat pile

In the case of a shoulder to head-high mat pile (depending on the height of the athlete), the step onto the mat pile with grip on the top edge can be supported by the free leg so that the hips easily clear the top edge allowing you to tuck jump easily on top or even over the mat pile (see photos 1-3, page 186).

Learning to dismount safely from the mat pile is an important skill that is easy and necessary to incorporate into the exercise program.

There is also naturally the possibility to finish with a drop with soft mats or a precision jump onto a longways horse. Mat piles are also easy to incorporate into obstacle courses.

ERROR CORRECTION

Observation	Cause	Corrective Action
The athlete slips down the wall.	His center of gravity is too near the wall.	Deliberately convert forward momentum into height.
The athlete pushes away from the wall instead of up.	The take-off is too far from the wall.	Take off nearer the wall.
The athlete reaches the top edge but not in a support position.	Lack of strength in the arms and torso. Pushing up into the support position does not directly follow the grip in the hanging position.	In this case, specific strength training is possible (e.g., dips, page 78). Practice fast Wall Runs.

© www.move-artistic.com

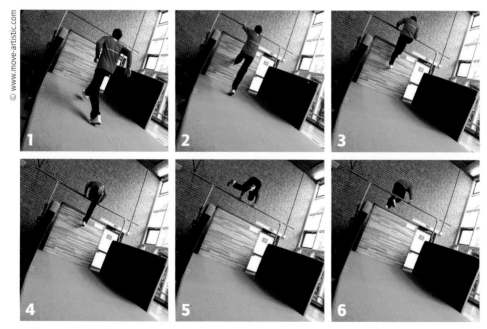

Wall Run – examples for apparatus layouts.

© www.move-artistic.com

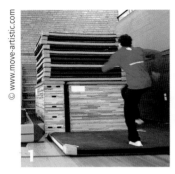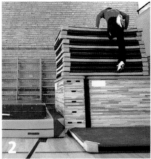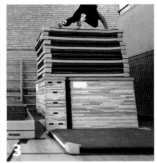

Wall Run – examples for apparatus layouts.

4.6.2 CAT LEAP/ARM JUMP – SAUT DE BRAS

Cat leap/Arm Jump is a **jump** with a **landing** in a **hanging position**, e.g., on a wall edge or a flat roof. This technique is used if it is no longer possible to land on the feet because the distance is too far or too high. From the hanging Cat Leap/Arm Jump position, one can either drop down to a lower level or push oneself up into the support position in order to reach the obstacle (e.g., roof, see final phase of the Wall Run, page 180).

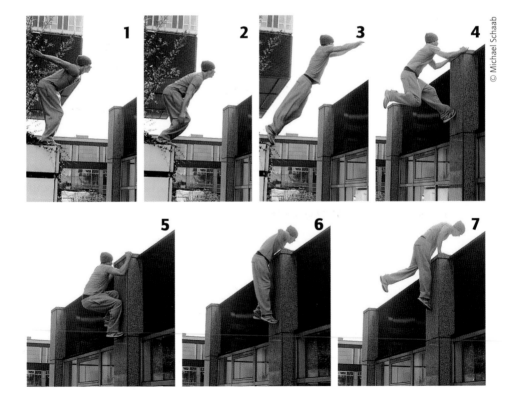

© Michael Schaab

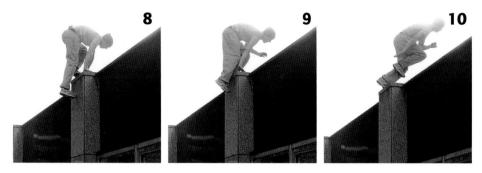

Photo sequence 31: Cat Leap to support and stand.

MOVEMENT DESCRIPTION:

Preparation

1./2. One or two-footed take-off from a running or standing start.

3. Fast, powerful body extension diagonally upward, the arms swing up vigorously forward toward the target.

3. Bring the legs up and forward in the flight phase.

Execution

4./5. The ball(s) of the foot/feet and the hands touch the obstacle almost simultaneously. The hands grip the top edge of the obstacle to stop you from slipping down. However, the farther the jumping distance, the more important it is to retain the momentum from the jump. The legs can land parallel or in a lunge position one above the other.

Landing

6.-10. It is possible to drop from this hanging position, however the skill is in pulling yourself up to the high level. As in the Wall Run, do this by pulling yourself up into the support position and then standing up (page 179 onward).

TIPS AND TRICKS

- *Before performing a Cat Leap, check the edge of the wall to avoid slipping.*
- *When you first attempt a Cat Leap, it is advisable to plant the feet one above the other against the wall so that one foot can quickly be put on the ground if you slip off.*
- *The legs should not be planted too high against the wall as then your hands could easily slip and you could fall onto your back on the ground.*

Variation

■ Level to Level Cat

Special Features

In a Level to Level Cat, the take-off is on the same level as the Cat Leap/Arm Jump landing. This means that you must jump down into the Cat Leap/Arm Jump position. This kind of downward trajectory means that the body must absorb more momentum with the hands, legs and feet when landing and that the feet cannot be optimally planted against the wall. If you realize this, you can simply let your feet slip down the wall and hang with your body straight from your hands on the top edge of the wall. This naturally means that it is harder to pull yourself up, but it does prevent a possible fall.

Nothing is impossible

■ Cat to Cat (from the hanging position [Cat Leap position], jump and make a 180° rotation around the longitudinal axis into a Cat leap position)

METHODOLOGY   *A. Outdoors*

LEARNING STEPS:

1. *Long hang on a wall*

   Task: Hang from an obstacle (top edge of a shoulder to head-high wall) with one foot resting against the surface/wall.

   Aim: Start off by getting a feel for the arm and finger strength required.

2. *Task: Stand next to a head to reach-height wall and grip the top edge with your hands. Then place one leg on the obstacle just below hip height. From this position, the upper body hangs with the arms straight. The second leg rests against the wall below the first leg.*

   Variation: 1-2 stride approach, take-off, grip the edge and then hang from it.

   Spotting position: A spotter can stand to the side of the athlete and, if necessary, secure his back and hips just before the hang (see Indoors).

3. *Jump onto the wall edge from an optimal distance*
   Goal: Jumping a greater distance and evaluating the strength required.

Task: The take-off point is 1 yard in front of the obstacle. Two-footed take-off, the arm action increases the momentum. Tuck up your legs and bring them forward. First touch the wall with your feet and then grab the edge with your hands.

4. *Loading Increase:* *With a short approach, one-footed take-off from the ground or from a low height.*

   Spotting position: *One spotter to the left and another to the right to secure the athlete's abdomen and back.*

5. *Final Form:* *Execution of the Cat Leap*
   Aim: *Clearing different distances and heights using the learned movement.*

Variations

- Vary distances
- Vary height distances
- With and without approach run
- Vary take-off heights
- Vary grip heights
- High jumps and drops to (tuck) pull-ups/hangs

B. Indoors

LEARNING STEPS:

1. *Knee hang on the wall bars – springboard combination*

   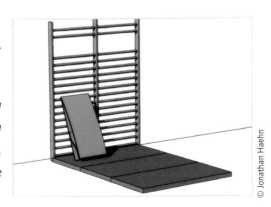

   Task: *Hang from your hands from the top bar, feet planted against a springboard resting against the bars, just below hip height. This position is the final position of a Cat leap/saut de bras.*

   © Jonathan Haehn

   Aim: *To make the final position clear.*

   Apparatus: *Springboard resting on wall bars and mats for safety.*

2. Approach, take-off into Knee Hang

Task: Approach run, then small jump into the final Cat Leap position.

Apparatus: See step 1.

Spotting position: One spotter can stand beside the athlete to secure his abdomen and back if necessary.

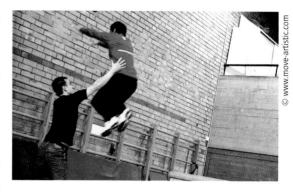

Securing abdomen and back

3. Take-off from box into Knee Hang

Task: Perform a Cat leap onto the wall bars from a small box.

Apparatus: Springboard propped up on wall bars and mats for safety. Small boxes or horizontal boxes as take-off aids.

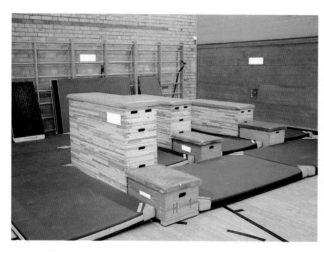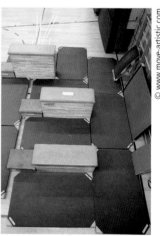

Spotting position: One spotter to the right and left to secure the abdomen and back if necessary.

4. Approach, take-off from a small box and perform a Cat Leap onto the wall bars
Apparatus: See 3.

Spotting position: See 3.

ERROR CORRECTION

Observation	Cause	Corrective Action
The athlete reaches the wall hands first and his knees hit the wall.	The upper body leans too far forward in the flight phase.	Compact jumping posture: bring the legs forward in the flight phase. The hands and balls of the feet touch the wall almost simultaneously.

© www.move-artistic.com

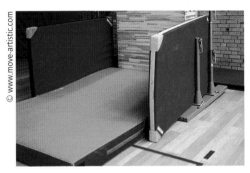
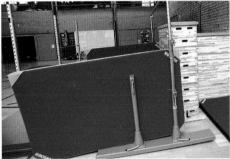

Cat Leap – Example of an alternative apparatus layout in the gym

© www.move-artistic.com

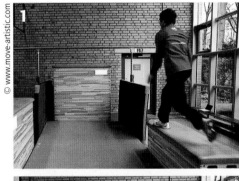
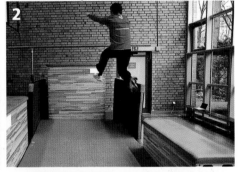
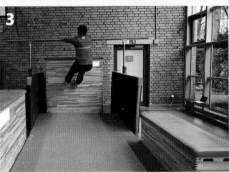
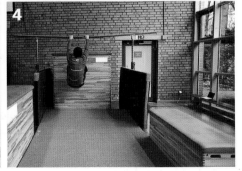

Cat Leap – Indoor photo sequence

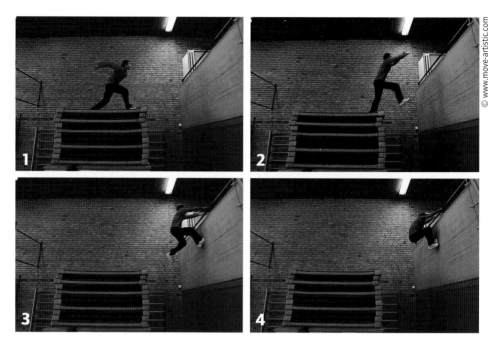

© www.move-artistic.com

Cat Leap – Example for advanced practitioners

4.6.3 MUSCLE-UP/CLIMB-UP – PLANCHE

The Muscle-up, called the planche in French, is a technique used to move from a hanging position to a supported position from which to climb onto the obstacle. This technique is less an efficient movement technique than an excellent strength exercise. In the city and countryside, there are only a few obstacles upon which it is necessary to perform a muscle-up in order to clear them.

An example would perhaps be a high ledge where it is not possible to perform a Wall Run up the wall. In the countryside, branches are examples of where one could go into the support position from a hanging position and then climb onto the branch. In most cases though, there are ways of getting around this technique and choosing an easier option.

The Muscle-up is nevertheless an excellent strength exercise that can add quality and speed to your Wall Runs, and you would be well advised to practice it.

The Muscle-up often seems impossible to beginners. However, with specific training, it is just a question of time before you master it.

Training Suggestions

- Pull-ups on a bar

- Dips on parallel bars

- Pushing up into the support position. From the support position on the edge of a wall, slowly lower the upper body (chest) onto the hands (push-up, see photo sequence 29, photo 10) and perform a fast, powerful push up into the support position (the legs hang below the wall and are not used for support).

- From the hanging position into the support position: from the hanging position, plant the legs against the wall (see photo sequence 29, photos 6-11). With support from the legs, perform a fast and powerful push up into the support position. Lower yourself slowly and under control into the hanging position and repeat.

TIP

Walls with a railing on top are most suitable.

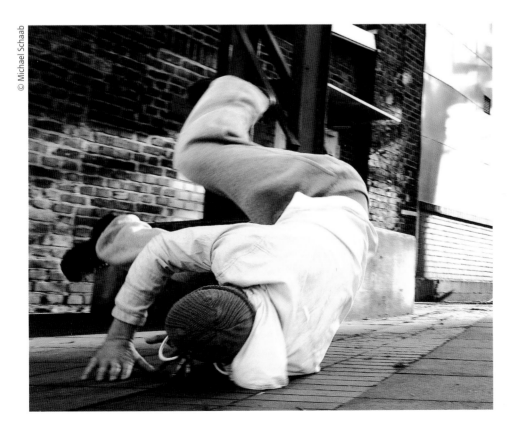

© Michael Schaab

4.6.4   WALL DISMOUNT

Safely dismounting from an obstacle is an important technique to learn, particularly for beginners. We humans, like cats, often find that it is sometimes easier to climb up than to climb down. If, as a beginner, you are still not used to cushioning drops actively in a way that is gentle on your joints, then climbing down is the only option.

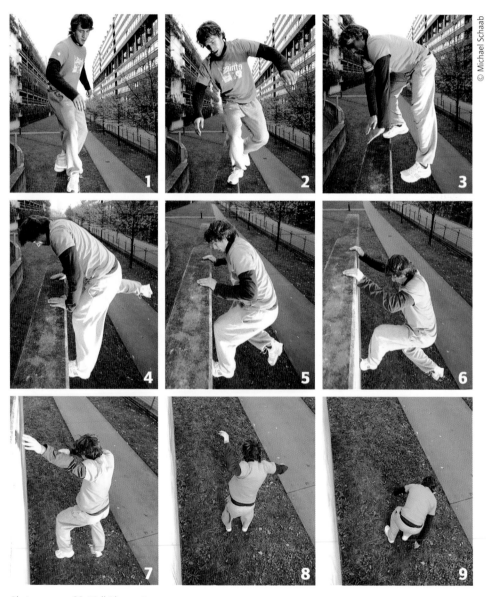

© Michael Schaab

Photo sequence 32: Wall Dismount

MOVEMENT DESCRIPTION:

Preparation

1.   From a standing start, look at the edge of the wall. Beginners can already drop down into the crouch position to make it easier to support themselves on the wall.

Execution, Part 1

2./3.   Rotate your the upper body as you look at the wall edge. Lower your center of gravity during the rotation and place both hands on the wall. The aim is to support yourself on both hands while looking at the top of the wall.

3./4.   In order to stabilize the support position, during the rotation, the toes of one leg (outside or inside leg) are placed against the wall, in order to control the lift into the support position. As soon as your feet move toward the wall, your upper body shifts forward in order to keep your center of gravity over your hands and to keep you from sliding off. If you have made it as far as the support position, then comes the hard part.

Execution, Part 2

4./6.   From the support position, move carefully into the hanging position. A Cat Leap position is a good idea (see page 186 onward).

Landing

6.-9.   Depending on height and experience, the landing is active into a standing position or with 180° turn in the direction of movement and a landing followed by a roll.

METHODOLOGY   *A. Outdoors*

LEARNING STEPS:

1.   Slow dismount from a hip to chest-high wall into the hanging position (same position as in the Cat leap, page 186 onward). On your first attempt, the wall should be low so that you don't fall far if you slip, for there is a risk of falling on your seat or your back if it goes wrong.

2.   Increase wall heights gradually.

B. Indoors

LEARNING STEPS:

1. Slow dismount from a mat pile

Apparatus: It is not always easy to construct a shoulder to head-high, stable mat pile with typical gym equipment.

Judo mats are the most suitable because they are firm and heavy and can therefore form a stable mat pile while also offering a firm edge to hold onto. The construction is really hard work though and should always be done as a group task.

Alternatively, the base of a mat pile can be built from 3 boxes, which makes it easier. It is also important that the mats placed on top, whether judo mats or small mats, have a relatively firm top edge.

Safety mats should be placed on the landing area at the bottom of the mat pile.

Spotting position: Secure the athlete on the abdomen and back in case of a fall when dismounting. The critical point is often when moving from support to hanging position, when beginners' hands can slip due to lack of strength causing them to fall backwards.

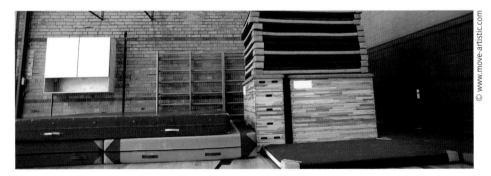

© www.move-artistic.com

Example of a mat pile

TIP

Mat piles can be used to practice more than dismounting. They are also a good way of introducing and practicing Wall Runs, Drops and Cat Leaps. In addition, mat piles are also easy to combine with other obstacles like boxes, horizontal bars or bars in an obstacle course.

4.7 HANGING AND SWINGING – LÂCHÉ

There are a few different hanging and swinging techniques in Parkour and Freerunning. Railings (e.g., in playgrounds) and branches are ideal for training.

LÂCHÉ

The French verb *lâcher* means **to let go or drop**. In Parkour, the term lâché describes **all techniques that start from a hanging position from the hands**. These movements are almost always combined with swinging movements, followed by a release and then swinging from another railing or branch or a release followed by a precision landing on an obstacle. Monkeys, who move quickly and precisely from one branch to another, are the ideal role model for these hanging and swinging techniques. Of course, we shall never be light enough to swing from branch to branch in the trees like monkeys can, however Oleg Vorslav has shown in his Internet video "Out of Time" (2009) that we can perform similar movements.

As well as good muscular development of the arms, shoulders and torso, these swinging movements with follow-up technique require excellent grip to get the timing right when letting go of the pole or branch in order to ensure a controlled trajectory.

In gyms, these techniques can be practiced with horizontal bars or uneven bars, and combinations of these apparatus often provide interesting and challenging possibilities.

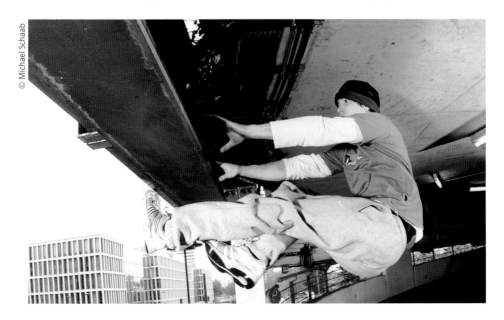

© Michael Schaab

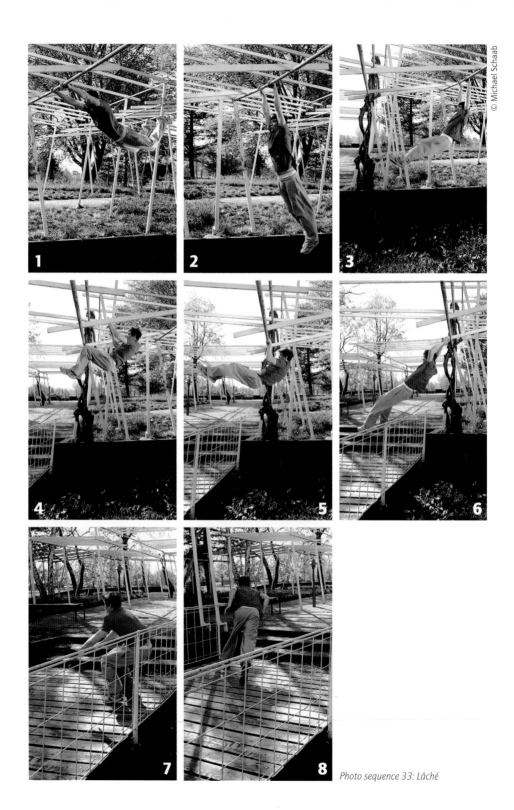

© Michael Schaab

Photo sequence 33: Lâché

EXERCISES FOR IMPROVING HAND GRIP STRENGTH

1. *Moving hand over hand along high railings / branches / wall edges / bars.*

2. *Swinging back and forth on railings and branches.*

TIP

Bend the hips for the upward movement, and extend the body for the downward movement.

3. *See above # 2, but shortly before the turning point from swinging up to down, let go just before starting the next swing.*

4. *Swinging back and forth then landing.*

TIP

Point your feet far in front to land.

5. *See above, with targeted landing on markings.*

6. *See above but land on box tops (placed horizontally).*

7. *From a standing start, jump into an elongated hang.*

8. *From a running start, jump into an elongated hang.*

© www.move-artistic.com

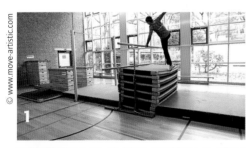 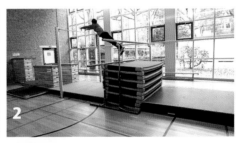
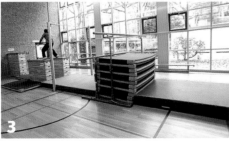 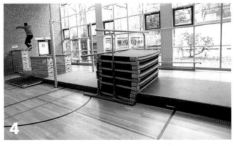

Hanging and swinging – example for apparatus layout in the gym.

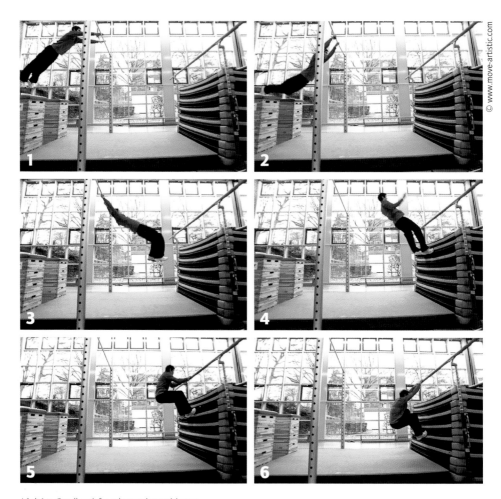

Lâché to Cat (leap) for advanced practitioners

4.8   UNDERBAR – FRANCHISSEMENT

The French term *franchissement* describes the technique used to jump through obstacles. Usually, this technique involves a railing, ledge or branch that can be gripped, allowing you to dive through between obstacles as flat as possible. This can be done feet, arms or head first. Here, we describe two movement techniques, the Feet First Underbar and the Spiral Underbar. As the core movement cannot be grouped with swinging techniques, it was not included in chapter 4.7 but both techniques have the same prerequisites.

4.8.1   FEET FIRST UNDERBAR

The Feet First Underbar resembles the classic gymnastics underswing, except that there is usually less room for maneuvering when clearing the obstacle, e.g., between two railings one on top of the other (scaffolding, climbing frames), in which case the Feet First Underbar resembles a Dash Vault (page 152 onward).

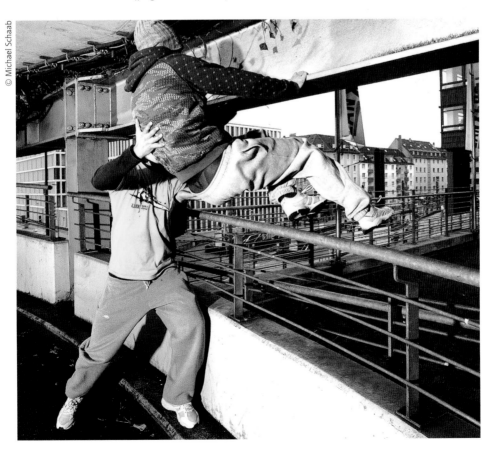

© Michael Schaab

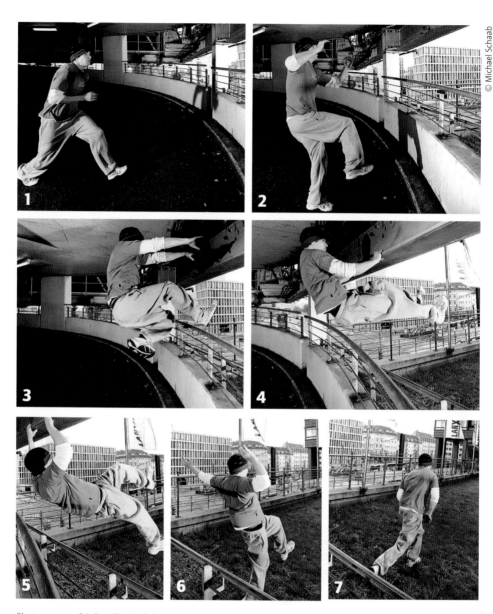

© Michael Schaab

Photo sequence 34: Feet First Underbar

MOVEMENT DESCRIPTION:

Preparation

1.   *Approach*

2.   *One-footed take-off*

Execution

3. The feet are brought forward so that they cross the obstacle first.

4. Grip the pole or ledge with an overhand grip.

4./5. The chest is brought up to the railing with a pull-up-like movement with the arms. Torso and abdomen are tensed. The feet are extended farther forward.

Landing

5./6. The hands can let go as soon as the head has passed the railing or when the arms are straightened again (creates distance).

7. Depending on the situation and follow-up movement, the landing can be two-footed or in the lunge position.

Combination

■ Underbar to Precision (Feet First Underbar with Precision Landing).

METHODOLOGY   *A. Outdoors*

Prerequisites

■ Jumping power and hand grip strength

■ Pull-ups

LEARNING STEPS:

1. Swinging exercises on a head to reach-high railing (page 199, exercises 1-3).

2. Underswing exercises on a chest-high railing (page 199, exercise 4).

3. Scaffolding or climbing frames are suitable places to try out the Underbar technique. The aim should be to clear a hip-high obstacle with the underbar technique. In the first attempts, it is advisable to place one foot on the obstacle to be cleared in order to push oneself over the obstacle. Once the technique has been well-tested, both legs can be brought over the obstacle together.

4. Aim for an Underbar technique in which you move from an approach run to a hanging position, then jog: approach, one-footed take-off, feet clear the obstacle first. The hands grip the railing in order to pull the upper body up. Land in a lunge position so that you can jog away immediately.

5. If you can manage this, look for a new challenge with a smaller gap to go through. Maybe you can even find a suitable tree.

B. Indoors

Prerequisites

- Jumping power
- Hand grip strength
- Pull-up
- Preferable: previous experience of the Dash Vault (see page 152 onward)

LEARNING STEPS:

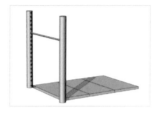

Preliminary Hanging exercises on the horizontal bar

The first two exercises have already been practiced on a head to reach-high horizontal bar in previous practice sessions.

Apparatus advice: The landing area is covered with mats for safety.

1. *First, swinging exercise on the chest to head-high bar.*
2. *Underswing exercises on the chest to head-high bar. From a standing position, overhand grip on the railing, free leg action and take-off from one foot in front of the railing. The arms start off bent but are straightened as you swing forward. Controlled landing!*

TIP

Think "feet forward." Keep your arms up.

First method: Underbar on the uneven bars

Uneven bars are suitable for the approach to the Underbar technique.

© (2) Jonathan Haehn

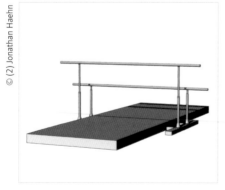

1. Swing up from hanging to sitting position

Grip the high bar with an overhand grip. After take-off, bring the legs over the lower bar (don't swing your feet out to the sides), thus enabling you to swing up into the sitting position on the lower bar.

Tips for apparatus: Set up uneven bars with the front bar set as high as possible and the rear bar as low as possible.

Alternatively, use two horizontal bars, one at hip-height and the other at head-height. Place small mats or a large sprung gymnastics mat on the landing area for safety.

2. Underbar with intermediate step

Task: Take off from a short approach; the hands grip the bar in an overhand grip and pull the upper body toward the bar while the legs swing forward. One foot takes an intermediate step on the rear, lower bar in order to bring the hips safely over the front bar. Release the grip to land behind the lower bar.

Apparatus: See step 1.

3. Underbar on the high bar over an elastic rope

Perform the complete movement over the elastic rope.

Apparatus: The rear, lower bar is removed and replaced by an elastic rope.

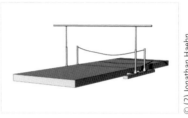

© (2) Jonathan Haehn

4. Underbar at the bar with spotter

Whole movement with spotter who secures the abdomen and back at the landing spot.

Spotter: The spotter waits for the athlete behind the obstacle and secures his abdomen and back (straighten up away from the bar).

Apparatus: Uneven bars where the front bar is raised as high as possible and the rear one is lowered as far as possible.

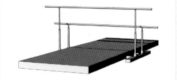

5. Target form Underbar on bars

From a running start, bring the feet over the obstacle, tucking the legs up. The hands then grip the bar for a brief hang, and the body extends in preparation for the landing, which is two-footed to start with, then one-footed then jog away. The obstacles become stable, higher and wider.

6. Movement connection

Running Underbar from running start while working on movement fluency.

SECOND METHOD: UNDERBAR THROUGH A HORIZONTAL BAR "WINDOW"

1. **Approach, one-footed take-off, landing in sitting position** *on a hip-high, soft pile of mats*

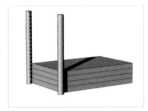

Apparatus: The mat pile should be at least hip-height, the front edge touching both bar posts (mat pile: 3-4 thick mats or a soft mat on small boxes or two thick mats on three parallel gym benches).

→ Compare method for Dash Vault (page 152 onward).

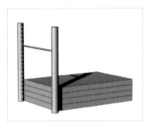

2. Underbar to sitting position

Fix a horizontal bar between the posts at reach height. Grip the bar just before reaching the sitting position on the mat pile.

3. Underbar over an elastic rope.

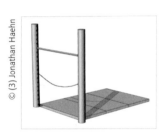

Mat pile Preparation: now use just one thick landing mat, but with an elastic rope stretched between the posts at hip-height. Approach, one-footed take-off and swing the bent legs one after the other over the elastic rope, then grip the higher bar with the hands. The feet swing into a two-footed landing (a one-footed landing as your confidence increases), releasing your hands from the bar as you do so. One-footed lunge landing, then jog away.

Variation

The elastic rope is stretched diagonally between the posts. The window to be jumped through is then narrowed near one post but still wide near the other. The runner decides which size gap he will jump through during the approach run.

4. Underbar over different obstacles

The obstacles to be jumped over are changed; they become "hard" and wider.

■ Place a gym bench parallel to and underneath the elastic rope (behind the post) and put a landing mat behind it.

■ Place two gym benches one on top of the other and exactly parallel and almost directly below the high horizontal bar (behind the posts out of sight of the incoming runner).

■ Small boxes and hip-high vaulting horses can be placed parallel to and underneath the top horizontal bar to be jumped over.

5. Underbar through the bar "window"

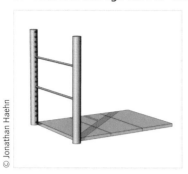

© Jonathan Haehn

A horizontal bar is fixed at least hip-high below the reach height horizontal bar (bar window). Run up and go through the bar window using an Underbar technique then jog away.

Spotter: The spotter waits for the athlete in front of the obstacle and supports him at the back, thigh and, if necessary, the hips.

© www.move-artistic.com

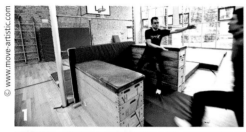
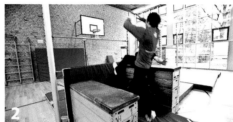
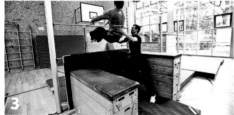
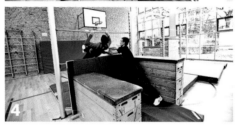

Advice on landing surface: The landing surface should at first be covered with thin gym mats. As your confidence increases, you can land directly onto the gym floor.

Extension: The size of the bar window can be reduced by raising the lower horizontal bar.

ERROR CORRECTION

Observation	Cause	Corrective Action
The athlete does not clear the obstacle.	• The athlete grips the bar first and the body and legs/feet lag behind. • Fear.	• First clear the obstacle with your feet, then grip the bar (methodical step: seated landing on mat pile or practice over a elastic rope).

4.8.2   SPIRAL UNDERBAR

The Spiral Underbar is a very versatile Underbar technique. It is mainly used if the bar can be gripped at head or reach height. In addition, it is a suitable technique for **clearing an obstacle** that is too far in front of the bar/railing/branch.

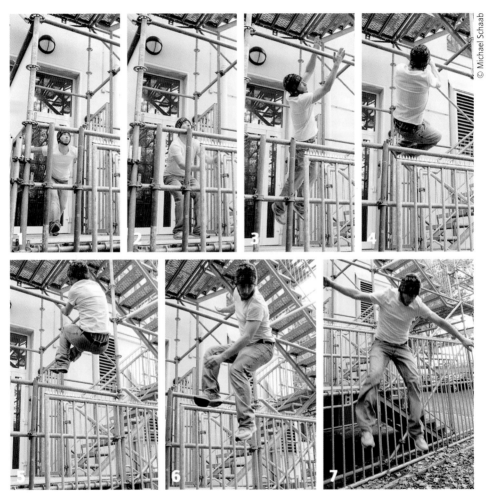

© Michael Schaab

Photo sequence 35: Spiral Underbar

MOVEMENT DESCRIPTION:

Preparation

1.   *Approach.*

2.   *Take-off can be one-footed, two-footed or from the lunge position.*

3.   *Lead with one shoulder and/or one arm.*

Execution

3./4.   The hands use a crossed mixed grip to grip the bar, with the lead hand gripping the bar from underneath and the rear arm gripping it from above.

4.   The head dives first under the bar, then the upper body is pulled toward the bar and the legs tucked up.

5./6.   Torso and legs are turned to initiate a complete rotation around the longitudinal axis. The hand in the overhand grip is first to let go of the bar.

6.   Look in the direction of movement; the lead hand now lets go of the bar also.

Landing

7.   The landing can be two-footed or in a lunge position depending on the situation and the movement that follows.

Combination

- Spiral Underbar to Precision.

METHODOLOGY   *A. Outdoors*

Prerequisites

- Jumping strength and good hand grip
- Pull-ups

LEARNING STEPS:

1. Practice jumping into the crossed mixed grip. It is best to use a branch or railing that is above head-height.

2. Jump into a hanging position with a crossed mixed grip, with pull-up and rotation around the longitudinal axis with the legs tucked.

3. Jump up to a railing/branch, running Spiral Underbar technique.

4. Only when you have mastered the rough form of this technique should you start to try the Underbar over obstacles. Start by using obstacles like banana crates (stacked up) underneath your railing or branch. Only after mastering that should you try to clear solid obstacles.

B. Indoors

Prerequisites

■ Jumping strength and good hand grip

■ Pull up

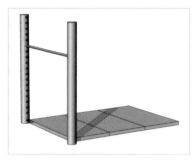

Preparatory hanging exercises on the horizontal bar

The first two exercises have already been practiced in the previous exercises on head to reach-height bars.

Advice for apparatus set-up: The landing area should be secured with mats (thicker landing mats if necessary).

LEARNING STEPS:

1. *Practice the crossed mixed grip on a head-high horizontal bar with mats for safety*

2. *Jump into the hanging position with crossed mixed grip, pull-up and rotation around the longitudinal axis*

    Tuck the legs up during the rotation.

3. *Spiral Underbar on the uneven bars or horizontal bars*

    Take a running jump to an over head-height bar or a horizontal bar with a crossed mixed grip, then perform a Spiral Underbar and jog away.

3.a The first step using the uneven bars is a Spiral Underbar from a sitting position. Sit on the lower bar with the lead shoulder pointing toward the lower bar. Then grip this bar with a crossed mixed grip and dive head first under the bar. Use your arms to pull your body to the bar with your legs tucked. Extend your legs toward the floor to land.

3.b Next, remove the lower bar and replace it with an elastic rope.

4. *Spiral Underbar on uneven bars*

    Only attempt the Spiral Underbar over obstacles once you have mastered the rough form of the technique. A suitable obstacle for use in a Physical Education class is the uneven bars, where the top

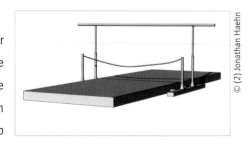

bar is raised as high as possible and the bottom bar is lowered as far as possible.

Alternatively, two horizontal bars can also be used with one at hip height and the other at head height. It is advisable to provide small mats or a large sprung mat to ensure a safe landing.

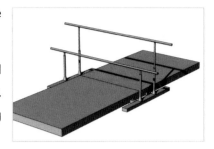

Another possibility is to use an elastic rope. The bar that is removed must be taken away (if necessary covered by a vertical mat). The aim is to dive over the elastic rope with the arms and head first and to perform a Spiral Underbar under the high bar. The hands use a crossed mixed grip to grip the bar, the head dives under the bar, while you keep your eyes on the bar and your abdomen pointing at the floor. The rotation around the longitudinal axis is supported by a leg tuck. Look in the direction of movement and release your rear hand from the bar. Land with your feet in a lunge position to enable you to jog away immediately.

5. *Spiral Underbar through bars*

Apparatus: See step 3.
Alternatively, two horizontal bars can also be used with one at hip-height and the other at head-height.

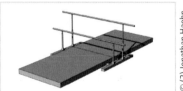

© (2) Jonathan Haehn

Error Correction

Observation	Cause	Corrective Action
The athlete sits on the obstacle.	• Pull-up action by the arms is missing. • The legs "hang." • The approach is too slow.	• Look at the bar, grip it and immediately perform a pull-up. • Tuck your legs up to your tummy. • Increase approach speed; don't slow down in front of the bar.

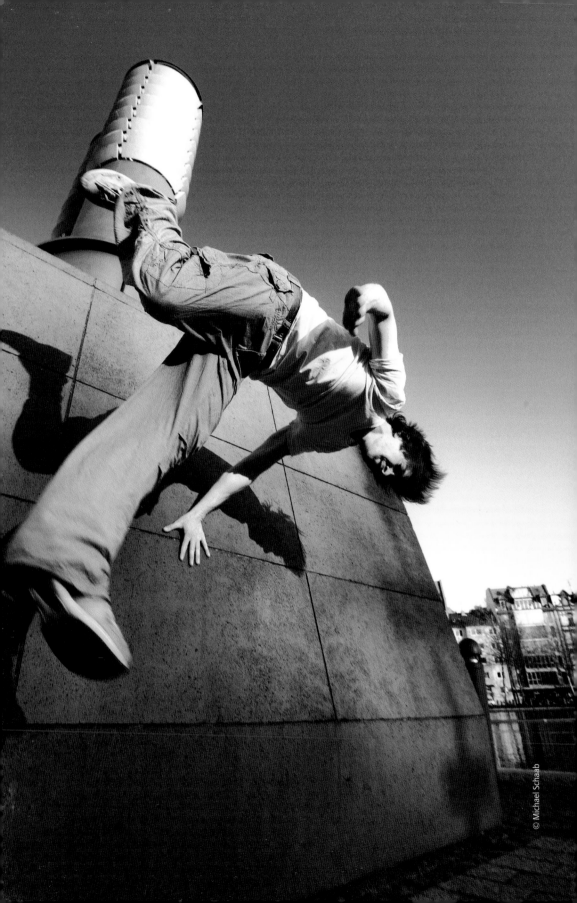

5   FREERUNNING - ADVANCED MOVES

Preliminary training in the gym with mats is advisable for acrobatic moves like those performed in Freerunning because it is very easy for beginners to seriously injure themselves on hard surfaces when performing overhead moves. That is why the advanced Freerunning moves presented here should be viewed as techniques for advanced practitioners and why in this book the indoor instructions are given first. Only once these moves have been mastered by regular practice should they be attempted outdoors.

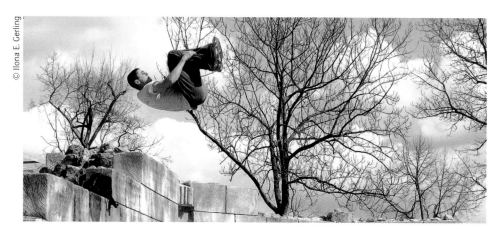

© Ilona E. Gerling

Front Flip from a wall – Freerunner. A'Bel Kocsis/Budapest/Hungary. Second place in Parcouring Competition in Berlin 2009.

5.1   LOOPS – CULBUTER

Tricks and Flips are often performed in Freerunning from heights, over obstacles or over gaps. This type of stunt requires plenty of previous experience to avoid the risk of serious injury.

As a basic rule, you should bear in mind the following maxim: don't perform overhead moves from heights onto hard surfaces until you have mastered the move on the flat or can perform it fluently with a spotter and safety measures. A Back Flip from a height certainly *appears* easier than a Back Flip from a standing position, but the forces that act on the body and the joints when landing from a height on a hard surface should not be underestimated.

If you can perform a Back Flip from a standing position, you can assume that outdoors too you have sufficient spatial awareness to be able to safely control the move and sufficient leg resilience to cushion your accelerated body so that outdoors you can also land from greater heights onto hard surfaces without injury.

If you progress to performing flips from heights during your learning process, look for a soft landing area, such as sand or a soft forest floor. For take-off assistance, you can use knee to hip-high objects like steps, fallen tree trunks, park benches or low walls as a step. In these initial attempts, a partner is also always helpful to provide support and/or security.

5.1.1 AERIAL

It is a really strange feeling to take off and swing your legs over your head and fly upside down. The good thing about the aerial is that you always have eye-contact with the ground.

Aerial is an unsupported free extended sideways somersault and therefore a 360° rotation. Its peculiarity is that (unlike the other somersaults or flips) you rotate around all 3 axes of the body: at the start of the move, your upper body rotates around the lateral axis as it drops, with the first quarter rotation the body turns around the longitudinal axis, in the flight phase sideways around the sagittal axis, then in the next quarter rotation again around the longitudinal axis and finally as the trunk straightens up, around the lateral axis again.

Aerials can be performed from a standing, walking or skipping start, from a combination of running and skipping, on the same level or from a higher to a lower level.

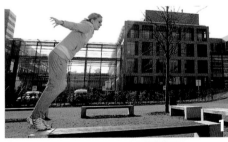
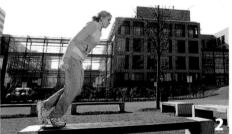
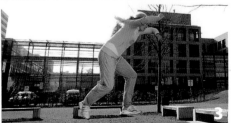
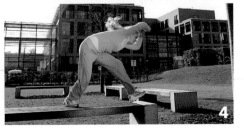

© Michael Schaab

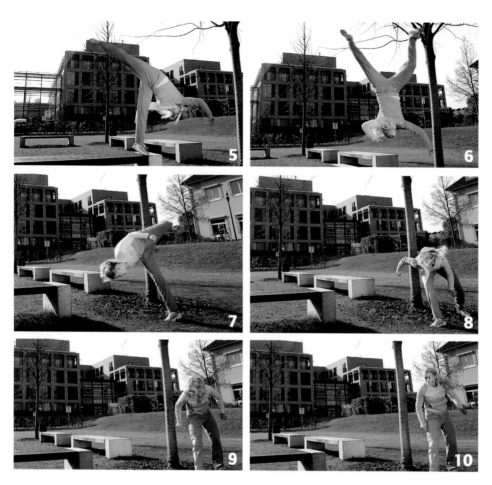

Photo sequence 36: Aerial

MOVEMENT DESCRIPTION:

Preparation

The preparation for the Aerial can be done in different ways: from an approach then skips, from a walk then skips, from a turn or from a standing start with a free leg movement.

1.   A preliminary movement.

2.   Bring the base leg forward and raise the arms diagonally forward.

3./4.   Bend the base leg slightly, followed by an active, fast and powerful lowering of the upper body forward to support the center of gravity, the arms swing down and the upper body and thighs are at a 55° angle to each other.

5.   Swing the free leg up and back vigorously, make a quarter turn with the upper body

and reduce the angle between the upper body and the thigh to 45°. The arms swing farther down and back and into the sides next to the body.

Execution

5.   While you swing your free leg up and back, the base leg straightens due to the push off action and for anatomical reasons due to the increased angle between the legs. The center of gravity (hips) is meanwhile shifted slightly forward vertically over the support point and the body starts to rotate sideways around the sagittal axis.

6.   With the legs in a straddle position, the body rotates in a high flight phase. The arms are held at the side of the upper body or by the sides. The upper body starts to rotate around the longitudinal axis.

7.   The free leg is pulled underneath the body.

Landing

8.   The free leg is lowered into a one-footed landing; the second, extended leg is held back and using the forces of gravity, pulls the body backward as partial mass over the new support point and the foot/floor pivot.

9./10. The trunk returns to an upright position and extends into the standing position with one leg placed behind the other. The bodyweight is then shifted onto the rear leg.

TIPS AND TRICKS

When performing an Aerial from a height, it is advisable to do a two-footed landing in order to spread the landing forces over two legs. If your attempts are still uncontrolled, there is also the danger of landing badly on an incorrectly positioned foot. The straddled legs also come together during the flight phase and may fall to the ground due to the hips bending if there is insufficient height.

Variations

■ Axe to Aerial/Reverse Aerial

Nothing is impossible

■ Aerial Twist

METHODOLOGY *Indoors/Outdoors*

Technical Learning Prerequisite

Fast, high, vertical cartwheel.

Basic Spotting Position

Standing on the side of the base leg, one spotter supports the Aerial on the ground by facilitating the push off from the base leg with the near hand on the hips to simultaneously raise the center of gravity. The far hand goes, if necessary in the second phase of the Aerial to the hips, guides the turning movement of the body and keeps the center of gravity high for the landing.

LEARNING STEPS:

1. *Developing a high, fast and powerful cartwheel on the ground*

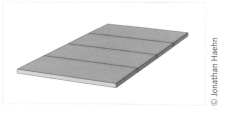

© Jonathan Haehn

Aim: Cartwheel on the ground, incorporating the performance-determining characteristics of the Aerial.

Apparatus: Mats

Tasks

Depending on your performance level, perform a cartwheel from a running start with skipping (for beginners), three walking steps (for very good gymnasts) or from a standing start with an introductory step (for elite-level gymnasts). With every run-through, try to incorporate a characteristic typical of the Aerial into the movement sequence. Don't move onto the next stage until the previous one has been mastered.

- Turn a cartwheel, aiming for a fast, head-on lowering of the upper body.
- Now quickly lower the upper body onto the front of the thigh and then make a quarter rotation with the upper body so that the second-placed hand is placed at right-angles to the direction of movement. Land facing the place you took off from.
- Turn the cartwheel as before with fast lowering of the upper body and delayed turning in, while trying to swing the free leg vigorously back and up to the ceiling.
- Swing the free leg up vigorously and make sure your front leg straightens.

■ "Now push off and up consciously with your base leg, aided by the action of your free leg. Now try to quickly and powerfully touch your upper body/chest with this knee, then quickly straighten your base leg knee."

2. *Basic Exercise: Cartwheel (Turn) into lunge position from a slightly raised platform onto a firm soft mat, sand or grassy field*

Aim: Introduction to the technical learning prerequisite for a high, fast "jumping" cartwheel, bearing in mind the performance-determining parameters (see instructions in the first task).

Tasks

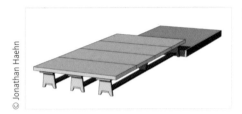

© Jonathan Haehn

■ The athlete stands on a long, slightly raised platform (Indoors: parallel benches covered with mats or two placed longways, two-part boxes = low box top Outdoors: bench with soft landing area and spotter).

From three approach steps, perform a cartwheel on the floor with support at the end of the platform then land. Following the bending forward of the upper body, the hands are turned as they are placed on the short edge of the raised platform so that the fingertips point back to the starting point.

■ In the attempts that follow, try to incorporate the typical movement characteristics of the Aerial one after the other.

Spotter: Sitting on the base leg side, one spotter supports the cartwheel from the platform by holding the hips (between abdomen and thigh) with both hands/forearms to facilitate the push-off from the base leg and at the same time trying to raise the center of gravity.

3. *Aerial with spotter's help at the hips and apparatus help*
Aim: Learn the support-free Aerial with help from a partner and apparatus.

Task: From three approach steps into a high lunge, perform the aerial with the idea that the movement will be carried out exactly as in the preliminary exercise, but the hands are placed on an imaginary extension of the platform – as if it were in the air. With the further exercise attempts, continue to add more of the movement characteristics practiced in the first basic exercises until finally the Aerial is performed successfully from the platform, even without assistance from a partner or coach.

Spotting position: One spotter on the base leg side places both hands/forearms on the hips, as though he were trying to scoop up the body, as though it were a ball in volleyball. As the athlete's skill improves, the spotter supports with just the hands instead of with the forearms. He lifts the athlete into the Aerial with his near hand, while the far hand holds the side of the hips and guides the body into the rotation. Finally, the athlete tries to land on his feet with no help at all. The spotter must often encourage the athlete by calling out, e.g., "hands up" to stop the athlete from trying to support himself on the landing area.

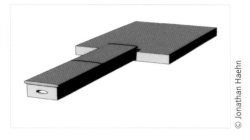

4. *Indoors: Aerial with hip support on the flat*

Aim: To perform the target movement with a spotter on the flat with a relatively soft landing area.

Task: Place two box tops horizontally one behind the other covered with a firm, thick mat. Exercise and Spotting position specifications as in the third basic exercise.

Apparatus Set-up Variations: A springboard with the flat side on a box top or a pile of four mats so that the springboard is horizontal. Walk along the raised platform and place the base leg on the side of the high springboard side to perform the aerial.

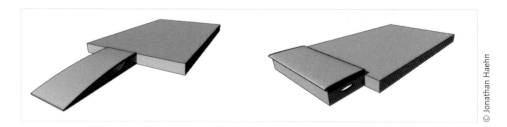

5. *Exercise to illustrate the free leg action and base leg extension*
A springboard or a 4-inch raised platform (indoors, if necessary, in front of a firm, thick mat) is placed at the end of the approach path.

After a short approach or walk, the base leg is placed on the end of the board/small platform. Because of the platform, the free leg has to take a longer path over the center of gravity. This forces the athlete to swing the free leg consciously and vigorously over his head and to push himself up high with the base leg. After this exercise, many people find performing the Aerial on one level much easier.

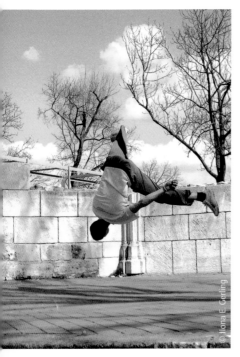

Budapest Freerunner

Spotting position: The spotter stands on the base leg side, one foot on the thick mat, the other in front of it, and helps the athlete at the hips (see above, if necessary, basic exercises 3 and 4).

6. Aerial on the ground

Aerial from a walk, skipping approach, or a standing start with one step into the move. At first, there is still one helper on the base leg side who with the near hand/arm raises the hips with the free leg action and base leg extension. The aim is to perform an Aerial without any help at all.

Advice: The hips can either be straightened or bent, depending on the individual movement style (see photo sequence 3, 6).

7. Aerial as a way of dismounting from a height

ERROR CORRECTION

Observation	Cause	Corrective Action
Rotation appears not to go far enough, landing on all fours.	• The movement is not performed fast enough with free leg action up over the head. • Athlete is not sure of being able to pull his hands toward his body or to the side when upside down.	• Perform a supported cartwheel with vigorous free leg action almost on the spot. • Repeated practice with a spotter, who calls out "hands up!"

© Michael Schaab

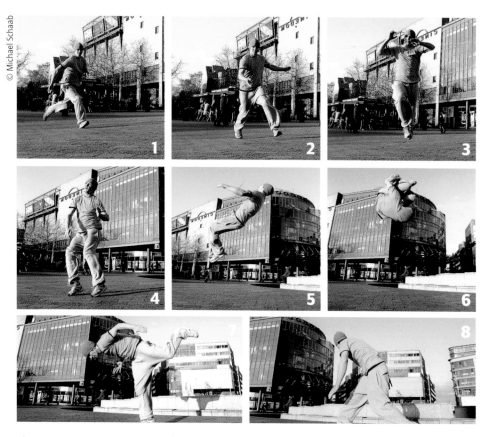

Photo sequence 37: Side Flip (individual style)

5.1.2   SIDE FLIP

MOVEMENT DESCRIPTION:

Set up

1./2.   Approach.

2./3.   Low jump into the movement, the feet are brought forward and land in a slight lunge position in order to achieve an ideal plant.

Advice: For a one-footed take-off, the plant is directly followed by the free leg action (see Aerial, page 214 onward).

4.   Sideways two-footed take-off. Upper body slightly turned toward the direction of movement. The arms are used as swing elements depending on the technique used in order to support the take-off movement.

Execution

4.   *Take-off.*

4./5. *Extend your body so that the front shoulder is behind the take-off point in the direction of movement when leaving the floor.*

5./6. *Flip around the sagittal axis.*

6.   *Leg tuck to increase rotation speed.*

7.   *Extend the legs out to the floor, but as in a traditional landing, bend the knees slightly. Keep your eyes focused on the landing area.*

Landing

7./8. *Two-footed or lunge position landing.*

Variation

■ Take-off from the lunge position with free leg action (see Aerial, page 214 onward).

Nothing is impossible

■ Side Flip extended with spread legs (straddle position).

TIPS AND TRICKS

■ *Tucking the legs up tight speeds up the rotation and allows for quicker landing preparation.*
■ *Gripping your legs allows you to tuck them up more tightly during the flip.*
■ *You should master the Side Flip before attempting the Flip alone on one level or from a height onto a hard surface.*

METHODOLOGY   *A. Indoors*

LEARNING STEPS:

1. *Learning the lateral plant step on the floor*

From a short approach, place the feet one in front of the other in a line so that you briefly adopt a lunge position (the rear leg is put down first) and take off.

2. *Introduction of a first rotation at take-off*

Approach, sideways take-off and landing on a pile of mats.

Apparatus: Pile of 3-4 soft mats.

3. Learning the flight phase and rotational acceleration

A pile of mats is needed to learn the flight phase with rotational acceleration by tucking up the legs. The problem beginners have is not turning upside down in the flight phase, but tucking the legs up in the flight phase and then preparing to land. In

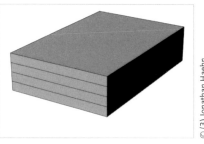

© (3) Jonathan Haehn

order to avoid injuries, we recommend a standing take-off from a long box (2-3 box sections) onto a trampette that slopes down toward a pile of mats. The take-off from the trampette is sideways to the pile of mats. The rotation starts at take-off and is increased by tucking the legs up during the flight phase. After the rotation, land sideways on the pile of mats.

TIP

If a fast rotation is followed by an uncontrolled sideways landing, the knees/feet may bang into each other, which is why we recommend sticking padding (e.g., foam) between the legs for this methodical step.

Apparatus: Knee to hip-high long box (2-3 box parts), trampette, pile of 3 soft mats and foam padding for the legs.

4. Side Flip over a padded obstacle with take-off aid

Apparatus: Lay a flexible soft mat or a firm block of foam over a long box. Lay soft mats behind it. If necessary, use a take-off aid.

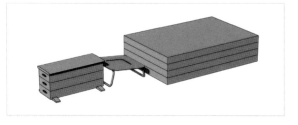

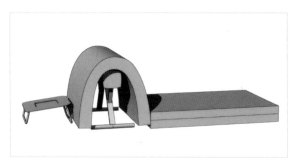

5. Side Flip with take-off aid and spotter onto a soft mat

Apparatus: Take-off aid (e.g., springboard) in front of a soft mat.

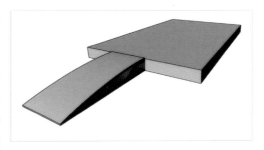

Spotter: The spotter waits for the athlete at the side of his approach. The athlete jumps with his back to the helper. The spotter's near hand supports the athlete's near hip and assists rotation. The far hand holds the athlete's other hip. The helper accompanies the athlete's movement with a twist grip into the standing position.

Alternative: From a height (also with free leg action) (see Aerial, page 214 onward).

Apparatus: Knee to hip-high horizontal box (three box sections) and a soft mat.

Spotter: Twist grip at the hips (see above).

6. Side Flip on flat ground with spotter
Apparatus: Mats

Spotter: The spotter stands behind the athlete's back to provide support on the hips during the rotation (see above).

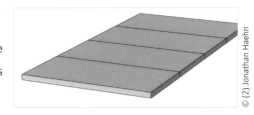

© (2) Jonathan Haehn

B. Outdoors

LEARNING STEPS:

It is much harder to learn Side Flips outside rather than indoors with mats and take-off aids. You should therefore be aware of a few steps in order to avoid injuries when learning.

1. *Side Flips into water*
2. *Side Flip from low height (or with raised take-off aid such as a rock or step) in the sand (later on grass) with a spotter.*

    Be careful in your first attempts, as when landing sideways, as it is easy to topple over to your side.

Spotter: The spotter waits for the athlete at the side of his approach. The athlete jumps with his back to the spotter. The spotter's near hand supports the athlete's near hip to assist with the rotation. The spotter's far hand also supports the athlete's rotation at the far hip or near the shoulder.

3.   *On one level with spotter (see above)*

4.   *Side Flip from height*

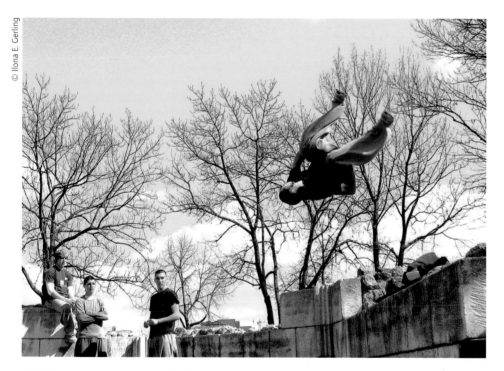

Side Flip from a wall – Freerunner from Budapest

ERROR CORRECTION

Observation	Cause	Corrective Action
The athlete does not gain height.	Often the result of an incorrect take-off plant is not caused by a flat jump into the take-off plant but an overly high one, which leads to a loss of momentum.	Flat jump-in, fast take-off (first practice the exercises on the floor without initiating the actual Side Flip rotation).

225

5.2   WALL TRICKS

Flips with sloping surfaces as take-off aids were already performed in medieval times (Tuccaro, 1599). These tricks were very similar to modern Freerunning Wall Tricks. However, since the origin of Freerunning, the variety of acrobatic tricks on walls has increased dramatically. Creative ideas and experiments are leading to the appearance of more and more new variations of these wall tricks. We would like to present two wall tricks that can be learned relatively quickly with a few instructions and some support from spotters.

5.2.1   WALL SPIN

The Wall Spin is a 360° turn on the wall around the sagittal axis where the hands touch the wall for support. The turn is overhead like that of a cartwheel.

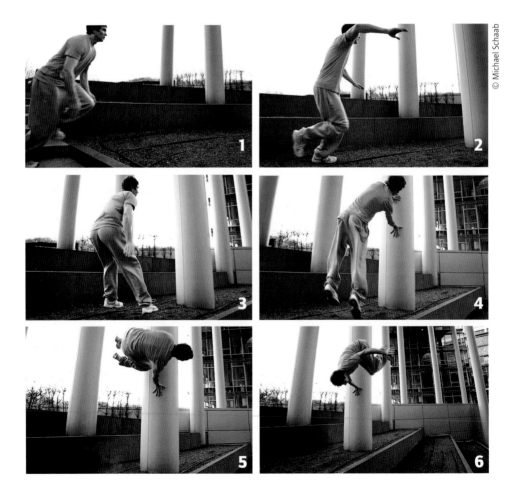

© Michael Schaab

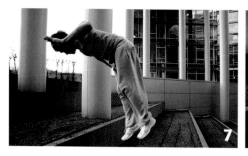 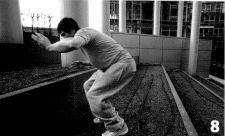

Photo sequence 38: Wall Spin

MOVEMENT DESCRIPTION:

Preparation

1./2.   *Diagonal to straight approach to the wall (about 45° angle).*

3.   *Two-footed take-off in front of the wall.*

Execution

4.   *Immediately after the take-off, place one hand higher than the other on the wall. The fingers of the lower hand point to the floor. The fingers of the top hand point in the direction of movement.*

5.   *The body rotates around the hands with the legs bent. The momentum should be provided by the approach and the take-off.*

5.-7.   *After one half of the turn, the top hand is removed from the wall so that the legs have room to carry out the second half of the turn. Keep your eyes focused on the landing area during the second half of the turn.*

Landing

7./8.   *Two-footed landing.*

Variations

- Wall Spin on a railing
- One Step Wall Spin (a step on the wall is used to gain height and to initiate the Wall Spin)
- Two Step Wall Spin (two steps on the wall are used to gain height and to initiate the Wall Spin)
- Corner Wall Spin (Wall Spin over a wall corner)

Nothing is impossible

- Wall Spin with one-footed landing and direct take-off into Gainer.

METHODOLOGY   *A. Indoors*

LEARNING STEPS:

Preparatory Technique

■ Palm Spin (page 172 onward)

1. Leg tuck and extension over the corner of a longways box

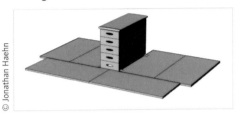

© Jonathan Haehn

Task: Stand facing the short side of the box, your hands grip the corners of the box, take-off and tuck up your legs with half turn onto the box. Straighten your legs again with a turn over the corner of the box.

Apparatus: Horizontal box (deeper than hip-height) with mats for safety around the corner to be used.

2. Palm Spin over corner of box (possibly with a spotter and take-off aid)

Task: From standing start, the hands grip the corner of the box, two-footed take-off, Palm Spin over a corner of the box.

Apparatus: Horizontal box (no higher than hip-height) with safety mats around the corner to be used (possibly with take-off aid in the form of a springboard). Apparatus see step 1.

Spotter: Half upper arm pinch grip supports the rotation by turning/pushing the hips (see photos 1 and 2, page 175).

Progression: With approach run.

Extension: In order to force the hips up during the supported turn, a light object (e.g., a backpack) can be placed on the box. The aim should be to raise the hips above the shoulders so that the movement more closely resembles the Wall Spin.

3. Trying out the target movement

Wall Spin to slightly sloping gym bench hung on wall bars or a box.

Task: From a standing start, plant the hands one on top of the other on a gently sloping gym bench. Rotate the hands as for a Wall Spin. After one half of the body rotation, release the top support hand from the bench. Look at the lower support hand as you move.

Apparatus: Hang several gym benches close together on wall bars or horizontal bars. If one end of the bench is higher than the other, remember to lay down small mats for safety.

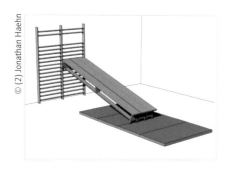

© (2) Jonathan Haehn

Progression: The benches are hung at progressively steeper angles.

4. Wall Spin on a slope with spotter

Task: Starting position: 2-3 steps away from the slope (inclined springboard). Diagonal approach run to the springboard, two-footed take-off in front of the inclined springboard, place one hand above the other on the springboard (fingers of the lower hand pointing toward the floor). In the support phase, turn 360° around the sagittal axis with the legs tucked, then two-footed landing.

Apparatus: The box is placed with a narrow end against the wall. Lay mats around the opposite narrow end. Lean a springboard against this narrow end of the box (place the wide end of the springboard on the floor, as long as the springboard has no rollers). This layout has the advantage that one can practice the Wall Spin without the danger of the feet getting stuck on the wall during the supported turn. The spotter can be introduced in this phase.

Spotter: The spotter's near hand supports the athlete's near hip by lifting and pushing, the far hand supports the rotation on the athlete's far hip or shoulders (see photos 1 and 2, page 230).

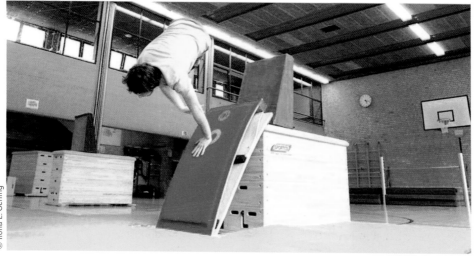

© Ilona E. Gerling

Advice: Bring your hips as far forward as possible.

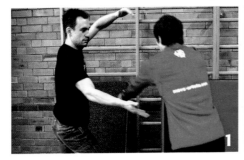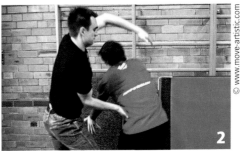

© www.move-artistic.com

Spotter supports the turn with a pinch grip on the hips

5. Wall Spin on the wall with take-off aid

1. Task: Reconstruct the support phase on the wall. Stand on the trampette in front of the wall and place your hands on the wall one on top of the other. The fingers of the lower hand point toward the floor, while the fingers of the top hand point in the direction of movement. Bounce slightly, then take off while leaning on the wall and

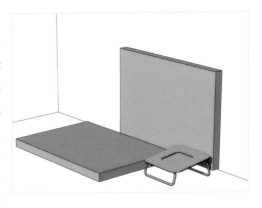

tuck your legs up then land back on the trampette again looking (to the front) at the wall.

Aim: Raise the hips above the lower supporting hand while leaning on the wall.

2. Task: Two-footed take-off from trampette, with support below the hips and initiation of rotation. The lower hand rests on the inclined springboard and the upper hand rests on the wall/soft mat. Look at the floor to prepare for landing.

Apparatus: Lay out sprung mats or small mats, use a trampette as take-off aid and a springboard resting against the wall to provide a sloping surface. For first attempts, experience has shown that it is helpful to place mats against the wall because the athletes' feet often slip on or catch the wall surface. They may also be afraid of the hard wall.

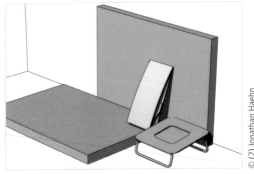

© (2) Jonathan Haehn

The soft mats should nevertheless have a very firm surface so that the hands don't sink in when leaning on them.

Spotter required! The spotter supports the rotation of the athlete's hips and shoulders (see above).

Progression: From a short approach, one-footed take-off onto the trampette then two-footed take-off from the trampette into the Wall Spin.

6. Layout of take-off aids

Layout: The trampette is replaced by two box tops side by side, which provide raised take-off help with a hard surface (closely resembling a take-off from the ground).

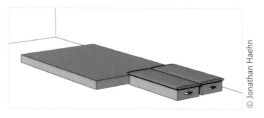

© Jonathan Haehn

The sloping surface and/or mat are removed from the wall.

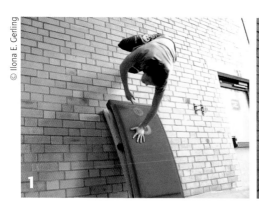
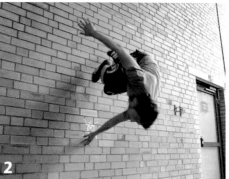

© Ilona E. Gerling

Later, the raised take-off aid (box top) is removed so that only the soft mat/small mats and the spotter remain.

TIP

As spotting gets very tiring after a while, especially with beginners, in school teaching or in training groups, the athletes should learn how to spot for each other early on! However, the spotter must be strong enough to lift and guide the athletes during the movement and stop them from falling. He must also behave responsibly, pay attention and concentrate.

B. Outdoors

The Wall Spin can be learned outdoors in gradual, methodological steps. However, there it is harder to find suitable aids, such as sloping surfaces.

LEARNING STEPS:

1. *Tuck and then extend the legs over the corner of a wall (below hip-height) (see Indoors).*
2. *Palm Spin on the corner of a wall (below hip-height) (see page 228), if necessary, with a spotter.*

Spotter: Half upper arm pinch grip and support the spin by turning and pushing the hips (photos 1 and 2, page 175).

Progression: With approach run.

Extension: To force your hips up during the supported rotation, you can place a light object (e.g., a backpack) on the wall. Try to raise your hips above your shoulders in order to more closely resemble the Wall Spin action.

3. *Wall Spin on a sloping surface (the flatter the surface, the easier it is)*

Starting position: 2-3 steps from the sloping surface, diagonal approach, two-footed take-off in front of the sloping surface, place the hands one above the other for support on the sloping surface. Do a 360° turn around the sagittal axis. After one half of the rotation, remove the top hand from the slope. Two-footed landing.

Spotter: The spotter's near hand lifts and pushes the athlete's near hip, while their far hand supports the rotation on the athlete's far hip or shoulder (photos 1 and 2, page 230).

Advice: Raise the hips as high as possible.

4. *Wall Spin on the wall with spotter (possibly with raised take-off aid).*
5. *Gradually reduce spotter's participation.*

ERROR CORRECTION

Observation	Cause	Corrective Action
The feet slip on the wall and may cause a fall.	Often fear of being upside down.	• Keep looking at the floor. • Repeat the preliminary methodological learning steps.
The athlete falls on his feet	The athlete is often not compact enough during the supported turn phase.	Increase rotation with fast, powerful leg tuck.

© Michael Schaab

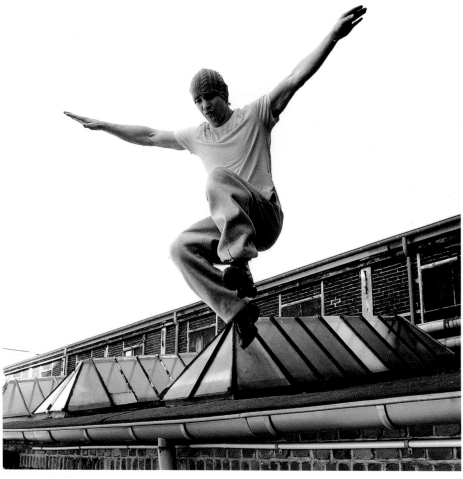

5.2.2 WALL FLIP

The Wall Flip is a back flip with one, two or more steps on the wall, which is performed by running head-on at the wall.

For beginners, it is best to start with the Two Step Wall Flip. Many beginners find this easier because the first step on the wall can be used to gain height and the second step to initiate the backward rotation.

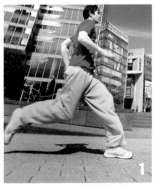
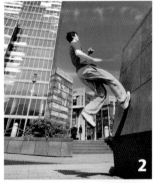
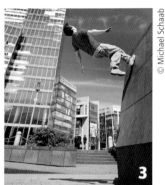

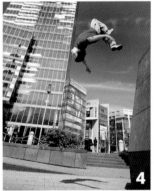
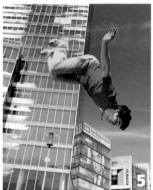
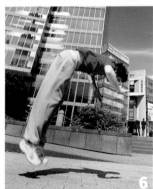

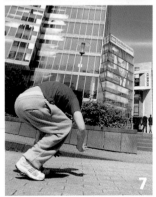

© Michael Schaab

Photo sequence 39: Wall Flip

MOVEMENT DESCRIPTION:

Preparation

1.Run head-on to a wall. Get the step in front of the wall just right (not too far away).

Execution

2./3. *Two steps on the wall; the first to gain height and the second to start the rotation in which you push away backward and upward from the wall.*

3. *Second push off from the wall by the free leg. The arms support the upward movement by swinging.*

3.-5. *The backward turn in the lateral axis takes place at the highest point by hyperextending the upper body backward, taking the arms with it and slightly tucking up the legs. This hyperextension enables you to see the ground more quickly.*

6. *The legs are straightened toward the floor.*

Landing

7. *Two-footed landing.*

Variations

■ One Step Wall Flip with the legs tucked, straight or spread out (Flash Kick).

Nothing is impossible

■ Wall Flip 360

■ Wall Flip 720

METHODOLOGY *A. Indoors*

LEARNING STEPS:

1. *Running up a wall and gaining height*

Task: Approach, take-off with the strong take-off leg approximately one leg length in front of the wall and two steps on the wall in order to learn and feel how to gain height. Concentrate on a controlled landing, looking at the wall. Don't lean your head back, but look at the landing area and keep your hands in front of the wall.

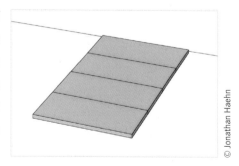
© Jonathan Haehn

Apparatus: Lay 1-2 large sprung mattresses or several small mats in front of the wall.

Consolidation/Variation

Approach, take-off in front of the wall and run two steps up the wall, 180° turn around the longitudinal axis, land and roll away.

TIP

To make the take-off easier, lean a springboard against the wall with the open side down.

2. Twisting over the head backward with twist grip help

Carry and twist away the athlete with the upper arm pinch grip (twist grip backward, see below) during the whole movement.

Task: The athlete takes a 2-3 step approach, takes two steps up the wall and tries to push himself up and back, tuck his legs up during the flight phase, and straighten his legs again ready to land on the ground and make a controlled return to the standing position.

Apparatus: Place a springboard on the mat and lean it against the wall.

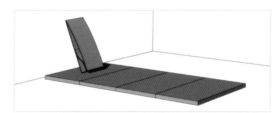

Spotting position: Two spotters stand side by side next to the athlete. They hold and secure the athlete with the upper arm pinch grip for the back flip.

- *The spotter should never let go until the athlete has landed safely.*
- *Both spotters must be strong enough to be able to hold the athlete.*

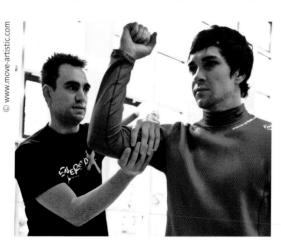

© www.move-artistic.com

Backward twist grip (upper arm pinch grip for back flip)

3.   Wall Flip with different spotting position

Spotter: Two people form a "lane" to the athlete's right and left. With the hand nearest the wall, they each grip one of the athlete's hands in a acrobat grip (the spotter's right hand grips the athlete's right hand. The thumbs of both hands wrap around each other). Now spotters and athlete run toward the wall together. When the athlete pushes off from the wall, the spotter's hand farthest from the wall holds the athlete's hips to support rotation in the flight phase.

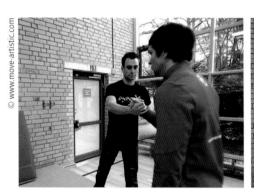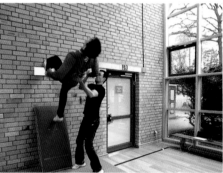

© www.move-artistic.com

The spotter's grip on the hand serves to stabilize the axis of rotation. The second helping hand raises the center of gravity and supports the rotation (two spotters are needed for this!)

4.   *Springboard as take-off aid is removed. Take off from the wall with support of the wall flip from two spotters with the acrobat grip and rotation support on the hips.*

5.   *The acrobat grip is kept to start with. The rotation support on the hips is gradually reduced until the athlete can generate the necessary rotation himself. Alternatively, the spotter's hand farthest from the wall can supplement the acrobat grip with a pinch grip on the upper arm.*

© Jonathan Haehn

6.   *When the athlete is able to perform the Wall Flip almost unaided, the last step is to completely do away with the spotter's acrobat grip support.*

The athlete now performs the Wall Flip almost alone, with the spotter just holding the athlete with both hands above and below the seat to aid rotation.

Spotter: The spotters form a "lane" and wait for the athlete at the wall. As soon as the athlete steps onto the wall, the spotters' place their hands farthest from the wall on the athlete's hips and/or lower back to lift him, while their other hands support the rotation in the seat and upper thigh area. The spotters secure the athlete's landing by holding his chest and back (the abdomen and back for girls/women).

CAUTION!

This security position requires a lot of skill and "quick hands" on the part of the spotters and should only be used if the athlete has already acquired a good Wall Flip technique and feels ready to "pull off" the Wall Flip unaided.

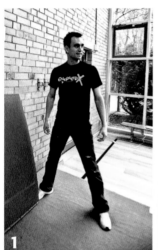 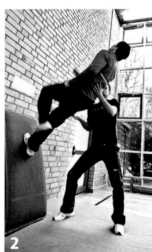 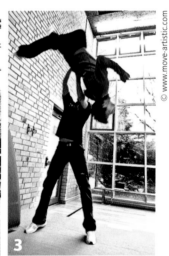

© www.move-artistic.com

7. *As a final step, the rotation support on the seat and/or upper thigh is removed and the Wall Flip is now only supported and secured by the spotters lifting the athlete's lower back.*

Spotting position: The spotters form a "lane" and wait for the athlete at the wall. As soon as the athlete steps onto the wall, the spotters' hands farthest from the wall are placed on the athlete's hips and/or lower back so that they can lift him if necessary. The landing is secured at the chest and back (for girls/women at the abdomen and back). This spotting position also requires skill and quick hands and should again only be used if the athlete has already acquired a good Wall Flip technique.

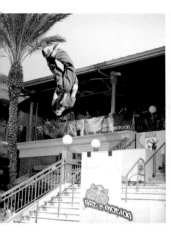
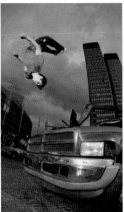
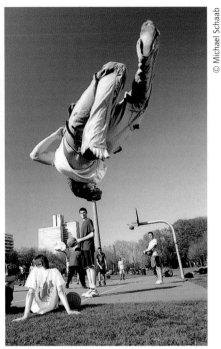

© Michael Schaab

B. Outdoors

Outdoors, the same methodological steps can be used as in the gym because the same spotting and securing support can be given. However, there are slight differences.

Look for a wall or a wide, high tree with good grip for your feet or shoes. A slightly sloping wall or tree facilitates the take-off. Ideally practice on soft ground as this makes the first steps to mastering the overhead movement easier. Both helpers must be strong enough to be able to hold the athlete!

ERROR CORRECTION

Observation	Cause	Corrective Action
The athlete rotates toward the wall.	The push-off from the wall is only upward and the approach speed makes the athlete rotate toward the wall.	Consciously push up and back from the wall.
The athlete falls almost stretched out onto the mat.	Open body posture during the flight phase, which causes a slow rotation.	Take-off upward and backward with hyperextension, then tuck the legs and bend the hips. Straighten the legs to prepare for landing.

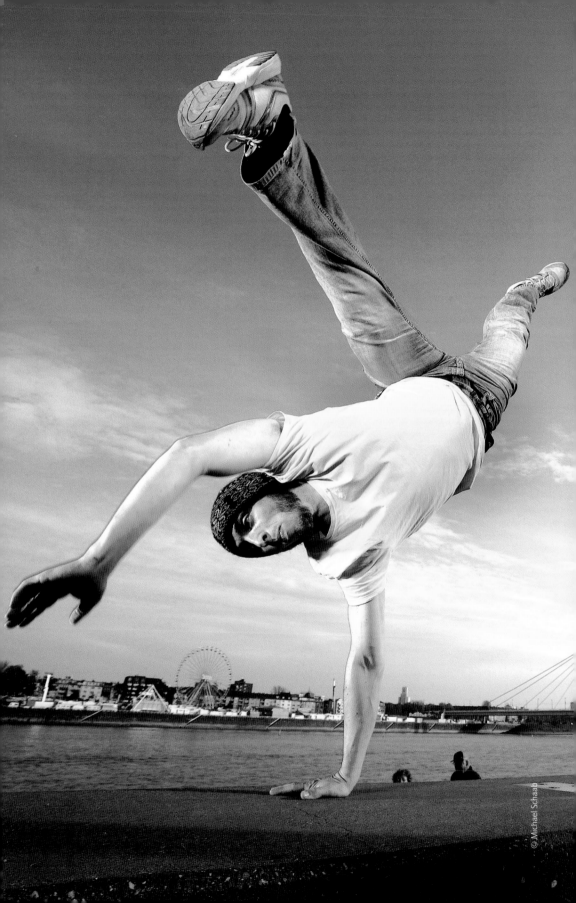

6 SCENE AND OUTLOOK

6.1 INTERVIEWS WITH SOME OF THE WORLD'S BEST FREERUNNERS AT THE ART OF MOTION IN SWEDEN

Below, you will find information "from the horse's mouth" about many top Parkour and Freerunning stars. Alex Pach met with the best traceurs and freerunners at a major event in Sweden in 2009 and talked with them about their thoughts, feelings and influences that make the Parkour and Freerunning scene so unbelievably fascinating.

You will get a feel for the two disciplines from the interviews and the insider knowledge of the movement arts contained within them.

Parkour is a form of movement that has been around forever and in recent years, has found new life in a modern, urban environment. All interviewees in this chapter describe their knowledge and above all the experiences they have had in and because of Parkour and Freerunning. They show us ways in which with these arts, or even sports, it is possible to make a living, broaden our horizons and redefine our goals. All interviewees mention a common theme: Parkour and Freerunning are primarily associated with the concept of freedom. The chance to develop as an individual is also a core message. Many of those I interviewed had already acquired basic know-how and prerequisites in various sports as kids that helped them get to where they are today.

They travel all over the world, get to know countries, people, new friends and cultures. They are booked to appear in international movie productions, commercials and huge shows. They meet with like-minded athletes from all over the world at major events or scene meet-ups and much more. They are living the dream!

In the tabular summaries of the interviews, you will also learn which dangers the interviewees think are associated with these movement arts, why injuries can happen and how to protect oneself from dangers and risks. This chapter also contains a summary and evaluation of the development of Parkour and Freerunning in the years to come.

Many thanks at this point to my team Daniel Borschel, Tim Hadler and Pascal Siffert, who provided help by translating my interviews. Unfortunately, I was not able to interview the best ladies on the scene, but would like to let you know that they do exist and in ever greater numbers. I hope you enjoy reading the summaries of the interviewees' answers.

**Markus
Gustaffson**
Helsingborg,
Sweden

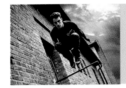

Gymnastics, inline skating,
skateboarding, snowboarding

**Khoa
Hynh**
Cologne,
Germany

Martial arts

**Gabriel
Nunez**
Los Angeles,
USA

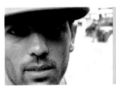

Gymnastics, acrobatics, martial arts,
soccer, basketball, football, baseball

**Shaun
Woods**
Sydney,
Australia

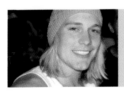

Basketball, soccer, tennis,
inline skating, skateboarding

**Ryan
Doyle**
Manchester,
Great Britain

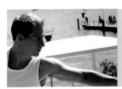

Martial arts

**Jason
Paul**
Frankfurt,
Germany

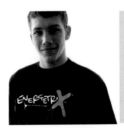

Handball,
martial arts, ball sports

**Tim
Man**
Helsingborg,
Sweden

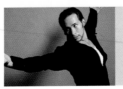

Taekwondo, wushu, capoeira
karate, jujitsu, judo

When, why and how did you take up Parkour/Freerunning?	Is it a good idea to have a background in other acrobatic sports (e.g., gymnastics, acrobatics, martial arts…?)
2004	Yes! Gymnastics is essential, but it's important to develop your own Parkour/Freerunning style.
2005	You start without realizing it as a kid (in playgrounds, in the schoolyard): you jump, hang, balance, climb... "it's in your blood."
As a kid, Freerunning after college 2001/2002 with *Jump London* (video documentary).	Jumping off cliffs and over benches as a kid, climbing walls.
High School, even before YouTube, I had seen various videos and just experimented with other people I met on Internet.	No answer
I was already doing the moves without really knowing what I was doing as they still didn't have names.	No answer
At the age of 14, I saw *Yamakasi* and tried it out with friends. First just Parkour, then with more and more creative elements from Freerunning.	No answer
Jackie Chan role model, Asiatic moves, desire to perform.	No answer

243

a) How do you train and

b) what do you think of competitions?

**Markus
Gustaffson**
Helsingborg,
Sweden

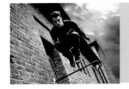

a)   Whether you train indoors or outdoors, the important thing is to know your limits.

**Khoa
Hynh**
Cologne,
Germany

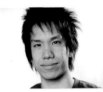

a)   Daily training, morning and evening.

Stretching, in-between strength training, technique training to consolidate techniques as every course is different.

**Gabriel
Nunez**
Los Angeles,
USA

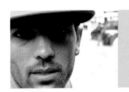

a)   Conditioning training, outdoor training, indoor training.

b)   I think competitions are good, as you can also match yourself against others.

**Shaun
Woods**
Sydney,
Australia

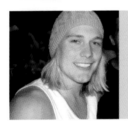

b)   I say "yes" to competitions! They look impressive, the atmosphere is great, friendly, community spirit, you can travel the world, good for the public to see such great practitioners in action. Important way of publicizing and drawing attention to the movement forms.

**Ryan
Doyle**
Manchester,
Great Britain

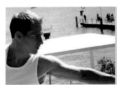

b)   Competitions are important to get yourself known, as that leads to lots of paid jobs.

**Jason
Paul**
Frankfurt,
Germany

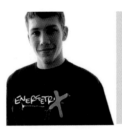

a)   Regular training

**Tim
Man**
Helsingborg,
Sweden

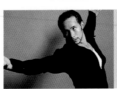

a)   About 6 hours every day, basic techniques regularly, simple but intensive.

Healthy training is important as I would like to do it for a long time.

a) Have you ever been injured and

b) what are the most common causes?

Which are the leading nations?

a) Dislocated shoulder twice.

b) The kids want to do too much too soon, try to do techniques that are too hard. Determination is often lacking (being afraid but jumping anyway).

England

a) Minor wounds, slight ligament tears, strains.

England, but there are also good people all over the world.

a) Just slight scratches, overstretching, back and knee strains.

b) Accidents: if moves are not secure and you overestimate your own abilities. The main issue is knowing your own limits so that you can reach or exceed them.

England, then France

a) A couple of accidents due to landing badly.

b) Usually accidents, silly situations caused by lack of attention but also if you are not prepared and hesitate.

Know what you are doing.

England

a) 2 broken knees in 10 years by landing next to the mat.

b) 50% mental strength. If you haven't tested the terrain beforehand.

England, Germany, Sweden and the USA

a) Broken arm when balancing due to lack of concentration, also 2 ligament tears during indoor freerunning training.

b) Overestimating your own ability is one reason, lack of concentration, coach's instruction leads to fewer falls but also less learning from falls.

I don't know, Latvia?

Not Germany, England has become strong but tends to include too much acrobatics and to neglect the typical Parkour flow.

a) Elbow, broken ribs.

b) Wanting to do too much too soon, hard techniques with too little foundation, not enough rest.

England and Russia

How are Parkour and Freerunning developing?

Markus Gustaffson
Helsingborg, Sweden

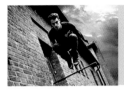

Possibly professional league championships, X-Games.

There will be stars of the scene, pros will do shows, movie stunts; groups will be able to make a living from it.

Khoa Hynh
Cologne, Germany

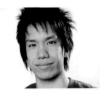

Hype, as there are already a lot of events.

Parkour will become as famous as skateboarding.

You will be able to make a living out of Freerunning.

Gabriel Nunez
Los Angeles, USA

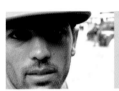

They arrived in the USA a bit later than in Europe

Used by the advertising, music and film industries.

The number of activities has quickly doubled and tripled.

Shaun Woods
Sydney, Australia

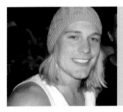

No answer

Ryan Doyle
Manchester, Great Britain

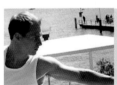

Everyone under the age of 15 knows about it, but the over-30s often don't. Big companies see the potential and could extend the profile of PK and FR further.

Jason Paul
Frankfurt, Germany

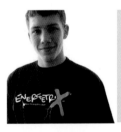

Freerunning is used by some as a way of being cool.

A decision must now be made as to whether the focus is on more competitions or instead on being together.

Tim Man
Helsingborg, Sweden

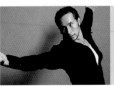

Very fast, from Parkour to Freerunning then more and more tricks, high level.

What is special about it, what motivates you and how has it changed your life?

It's my passion, my life. I am happy to be able to do it, for me it's the coolest thing.

Freedom and individuality. Unmovable obstacles, overcoming things with your own body.
Creativity is a motivation.
The euphoria when you pull something off, you feel free and unbelievably inspired, but also under control.
Training with other is motivating. Stars like Jackie Chan, Jet Li are role models.

It's a liberating feeling to see an obstacle that you think you can't clear, trying it and then finding you can do it. Competitions motivate me because I want to measure myself against others, as you don't need anything else except your body.

No answer

Individual style, I don't want to be the next Jackie Chan, I am the only Ryan Doyle.
It is more a philosophy, a belief in a destiny.
Life has a plan; you should take life as it is.

There are strengths; learn to challenge yourself; discipline helps you to be a good person, setting yourself problems; creativity; motivating the people you meet; places that you see; styles that you learn (from others or even from animals); always looking for new challenges and setting them for yourself; a new way of looking at the city and architecture; I have changed; I do strength training; eat more healthily and want to perform well; you travel, meet people; and it makes you more tolerant and open to new things.

Self-motivation comes out of the movement itself, also because the scene has become more interesting.
I like to watch it. I have been doing it all my life and am grateful for that and love my life.

Which companies or films do you know of that use this subject?

Markus
Gustaffson
Helsingborg,
Sweden

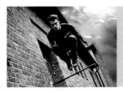

Barclaycard World Championships

UK will probably go to America, Red Bull, Art of Motion, K-Swiss shoes, Five Ten, Puma, shoe manufacturer Kalenjis ...could even become Olympic.

Khoa
Hynh
Cologne,
Germany

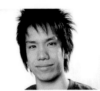

Dissemination on Internet, YouTube. Gatherings at which one can get to know the scene and swap ideas.

Barclaycard World Championships, Red Bull, Art of Motion, Kalenjis and K-Swiss

Gabriel
Nunez
Los Angeles,
USA

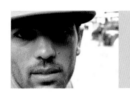

Workshops and events, e.g., Parkour Generation, Barclaycard World Championships, Red Bull contest, shoes like K-Swiss, Kalenjis, Five Ten ...more and more movie stunts.

Shaun
Woods
Sydney,
Australia

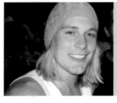

Kalenjis, Gingees

Ryan
Doyle
Manchester,
Great Britain

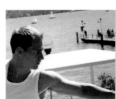

MTV Production Parkour Challenge, Red Bull Events, Films and Stunts, TV, Internet, dissemination on YouTube, Kalenjis (light and cheap), Puma (trying to get a foothold), K-Swiss (not ideal and expensive), Five Ten.

Jason
Paul
Frankfurt,
Germany

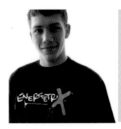

Playstation workshops and other scene meet-ups, internet forums and YouTube (caution: may be dangerous for beginners) are the information platforms, K-Swiss, Kung-Fu shoes are light and have grip.

Tim
Man
Helsingborg,
Sweden

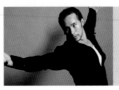

Many tricks and stunts in movies, so it's motivation for traceurs and freerunners. I have worked mainly in Asia. That's where most of the productions were that I was able to take part in.

Which message would you like to give the world?

Take it slowly! Safety first!

Fun is the most important thing!
Go through the world with a smile!
Always have a good pair of shoes with you!

Be real!
Be free!
Go for it! Just take everything that comes your way!

Watch less YouTube! Copy less and try stuff out more!
Develop your personal style!
There is no right or wrong, just what is right for you.
Be creative!

Individual style, I don't want to be the next Jackie Chan, I am the only Ryan Doyle.
It is more a philosophy, a belief in a destiny.
Life has a plan; you should take life as it is.

Don't get hung up on YouTube! Get out and move!

Practice Parkour as your concentration will improve, you will be more balanced, healthy and strong and so avoid injuries.

6.2 THE SCENE

Parkour and Freerunning are developing in a different way than previous trend sports, and above all, much quicker. PK & FR are communicated and brought alive by the new Internet media. YouTube, Vimeo, Twitter, Facebook, MySpace and other social networking sites contribute to the dissemination of information, and especially of images and videos. People swap ideas on forums and become part of communities. Thanks to this development and the associated target-group specific response to fans and the scene, organizations and companies are increasingly focusing on the topic and new markets are springing up which allow traceurs or freerunners to make a living.

Parkour as a traditional and original movement form still exists but is increasingly being caught up by Freerunning, which is becoming even stronger and is often still (wrongly) called PK. There are also new trends and developments in the PK scene.

The Parkour scene remains true to its original philosophy and still uses movement according to the guiding principles of David Belle (see definition, page 26). There are more trends in Freerunning though, which are emerging right now. First of all, there is the creative and playful branch, which can be seen as a progression from Parkour and still retains much of the element of efficient, purposeful movement. It has similar motivations to those of PK.

A second branch is that of the New Generation, who perform unbelievably difficult power moves with and around the terrain, using more and more techniques from tricking or classic acrobatics without obstacles. The trend here is often the difficulty of the moves or the presenting of new tricks on Web2.0 and other channels. There is yet another scene that swaps ideas and goes to jams, gatherings and other events to meet up in order to have fun practicing PK & FR.

6.3 GROUPS

There are numerous groups all over the world. I would like to just discuss the best known ones here. Alongside hundreds of teams, there are also professional organizations in different countries that contribute to the professionalization of PK & FR, to raising their profile and naturally also to the economic side. Yamakasi is not only the most famous group but also the first to be popularized in the media.

Urban Freeflow and *Parkour Generation* are two big names in Europe (UK). England is now considered to be one of the leading nations PK right now. In Germany, *Pawa* and *Move Artistic* were the first organizations, and others have followed suit. The World Freerunning Parkour Federation (WFPF), a partnership of some of the world's biggest names in Parkour, has developed as a major force in the USA and all over the world following its successful series MTV's ULTIMATE PARKOUR CHALLENGE. As a global community, WFPF is dedicated to the safe and respectful advancement of the Parkour Movement throughout the world.

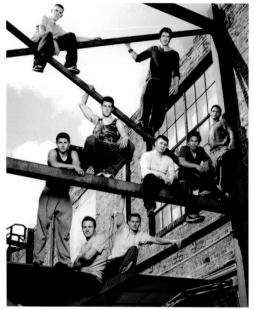

© WFPF

6.4 WORKSHOPS

Workshops are a good starting point for PK & FR. Especially for beginners and newcomers, but also for experienced practitioners, they offer the opportunity to get advice and tips from other coaches. Workshops vary greatly in what they offer. They range from those with absolutely no sport science content to perfect methodological-didactic teaching and learning of specific content.

6.5 TRAINING AND FURTHER EDUCATION

Until now, there has been no sufficiently well-founded qualification process for those interested in practicing and coaching Parkour and Freerunning in these still-young subject areas. There is also increasing demand for further training for teachers.

Some brave self-taught souls have learned movement skills by themselves using the Internet. They have acquired apparent expertise, however, without having learned the whole movement. The transfer of learning to schools, clubs and other organizations is also rudimentary as appropriate teaching concepts have not yet been fully developed.

We wish that more people felt competent enough to lead groups and advanced training courses. This would spread the growth of these great and complex sports. However, we are concerned about the physical and mental health of the kids, young people and young adults who are vulnerable due to an incorrect approach, giving rise to injuries or decreased motivation when they grow older.

6.6 COMPETITIONS

There are a handful of big competitions in the Freerunning scene, organized not by the scene itself but by industry or other agencies. However, experienced teams always have an advisory role in the organization of these events, thus lending them credibility and above all more security. Competitions are not viewed positively by all practitioners though, so there are two camps worldwide – those who are for and those against competitions.

Europe is not only the birthplace of the art of movement, but also the location of the first competition on the scene. The Art of Motion, sponsored by Red Bull in Vienna and Sweden (other countries will follow), the Barclaycard World Championships, as well as the Parcouring World Championships and the MTV Parkour Challenge as a broadcasting format are currently the biggest events. The USA is sure to overtake this in the near future thanks to its athletes and relevant business know-how, and the Asian and Russian markets should not be underestimated. Regional competitions also exist.

6.7 CLOTHING AND SHOES

Clothing plays a major role in Parkour and Freerunning, but this is as yet unaccepted/ exploited by the scene. In order to move, you just need a pair of good shoes, which don't always need to be expensive, but the brand names are also trying to exploit the youthful images of original moves and are developing apparently special shoes for the traceur or freerunner with varying degrees of success. Clothing and shoes must always, like your movements, be efficient, they must not get in the way or weigh you down. They should be adapted to the weather and be quite hard-wearing, however expensive items are often avoided. In the future, manufacturers will definitely find their market here though and develop special products for the scene.

6.8   MISCELLANEOUS

There are of course pros and cons associated with this rapid growth that are indirectly alluded to in interviews. Many beginners find it hard to know which of the many experts on the World Wide Web to look to for their information and above all for competent knowledge of the movement arts and how to perform them. Videos with homemade tutorials encourage you to copy and contribute significantly to learners overestimating their own abilities. There are, however, good examples of experienced practitioners and teams that have practiced for many years in order to pass on their knowledge as true experts.

It is certainly a good thing to swap ideas and suggestions with other participants and also to be connected with other countries or even other continents in order to keep in touch with current developments, but you should also listen to your natural instincts, have a little more respect for your health and environment and not throw yourself into a reckless movement through the blind desire to move or because of encouragement by other people. You should be prepared to accept new challenges. That means specifically conducting preparation of all the structures of your body for the coming stress and only then daring to take the leap.

The scene is also developing in a wider area toward professionalism and countless traceurs and freerunners are already making a living from their movement art. There are more and more markets in which one can work with PK & FR, although not necessarily as an active athlete.

In addition to the pros who scoop their titles in major international FR Contests and then go on to be in the spotlight in advertising, photo shoots, movies or shows, there is also a job market in the area of training and coaching. Pure PK and FR Schools and centers offer regular training courses and other events.

So this is no longer just a fringe phenomenon with crazy people jumping from rooftops; it is developing into a real industry. Event managers with specialist knowledge are needed to satisfy the demand for a wide range of events. Camera and video professionals, who understand something of the movements, are certainly another current example of a possible area of employment, even if this is not a full-time job. This is also the obvious place to raise the issue of authenticity and how the content and actual concept of PK and FR are to be portrayed. But with this it becomes all the more important that those who are active in these areas of work know what they are doing and have experienced, or are still experiencing, the movement arts first-hand.

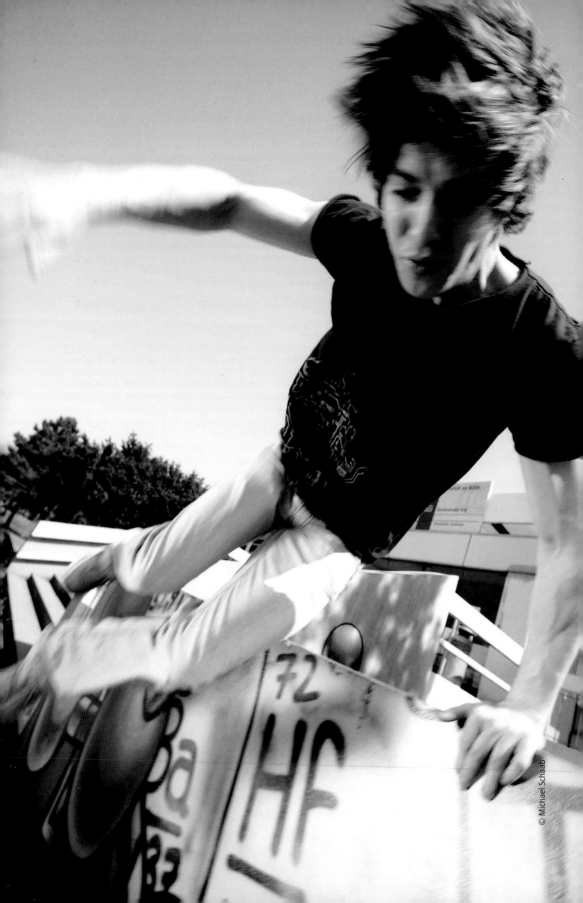

7   PARKOUR AND FREERUNNING IN SCHOOLS

This book is primarily written for newcomers to the scene of traceurs and freerunners. However, we would also like to devote a chapter to Parkour in schools, with a few tips, as it is enjoying increasing popularity there.

Even though the teaching of Parkour and Freerunning in schools may be frowned upon by the PK & FR scene, this is an unstoppable trend. It is a development that the pupils themselves have taken into the schools. Young people discovered it mainly on the Internet, tried out what they saw in the video clips and developed it into *their* leisure sport.

Schools would be foolish not to be aware of their pupils' current interests, and incorporate them into an educational and instructional physical education program. The Parkour scene should, on the contrary, be glad that its movement(s) are (will be) taken so seriously. The schools can provide them with countless new supporters, whether as active practitioners or fans.

In the Netherlands, a guiding principle of the physical education curriculum is *"participation in the movement culture."* The educational aim is that the school sports curriculum should include extracurricular movement cultures. Parkour and Freerunning belong to the new movement culture of young people.

7.1   PEDAGOGICAL AIMS AND RATIONALES FOR PARKOUR IN SCHOOLS

The physical education curriculum may be based on the six sports pedagogical aims identified by Dr. D. Kurz of the University of Bielefeld, Germany (see figure 14, page 258).

1.   Performance (competition, success)
2.   Excitement/play (risk, adventure)
3.   Sensation (physical experience)
4.   Health (fitness, well-being)
5.   Expression (display, creation)
6.   Cooperation (learning to socialize, environment)

The *six core pedagogical areas* are explored in the following.

1. PERFORMANCE

The decline in the physical ability of children and young people has long been a point of concern and is on the rise. Effort and performance should be reinstated as sports pedagogical categories and no longer neglected.

The significance of the performance aspect

- The promotion of readiness to learn and achieve

Positive attitude to effort:

- Parkour and Freerunning accentuate completely naturally the performance aspect by "persistent, repeated practice"
- Parkour and Freerunning allow for individual performance progression

2. ADVENTURE – RISK – EXCITEMENT

Adventure and risk are above all seen *consciously* by the teacher; the pupil *feels* only excitement, a kick, butterflies in his stomach. Young people are now looking increasingly for **authentic experiences** in the virtual world that determines their leisure time. Being in touch with reality means being in touch with oneself and one's body.

The skills to deal with adventure and risk are developed by Parkour and Freerunning.

Aspects of adventure and responsibility:

- **Enabling the perception and evaluation** of one's own abilities and limits in **challenging situations** with an uncertain (but secured) outcome.
- Introduction to conscious, prudent, **responsible** handling of challenging situations; learning to take **responsibility** for oneself.
- Development of a realistic **self-assessment** and a healthy **self-confidence**.
- Acknowledging **fear** and overcoming it.
- Formation of **a sense of responsibility** and **trust** in fellow pupils (when learning elements with spotting and securing).

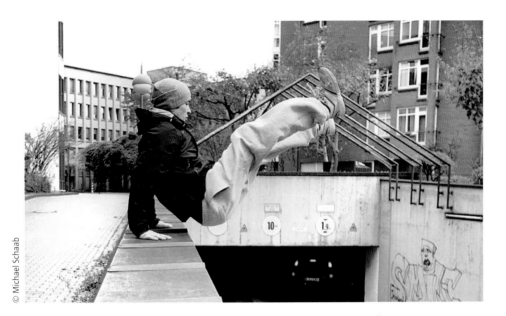

© Michael Schaab

3. SENSATION OR PHYSICAL EXPERIENCE

Aspects of sensation:

- **Movement experiences should be created**
- **Perceptual capacity** of all the senses should be improved
- **Physical experiences** should be extended
- PK & FR open up possibilities for creative physical movement
- PK & FR provide an inexhaustible variety of movement situations, tasks and solutions to provide opportunities for diverse movement experiences with all the senses

4. HEALTH & FITNESS

Aspects of health and fitness:

- Promote health and **fitness**, develop an **awareness of health**
- Improve **well-being** and form a positive self-image
- Optimize physical **performance ability** and mental and physical **resilience**

5. EXPRESSION

Aspects of expression:

- **Physical self-expression**
- **Structuring movement**
- **Playing**

PK & FR offer a variety of opportunities for individual physical self-expression and experience by

- **Playing** with movement/one's body
- Production of **movement ideas**
- **Performing and presenting** of movement ideas (video clips)

6. Cooperation and Fairness – cooperation and communication (competition)

- PK & FR offer very good opportunities in the working of stunts and tricks in school, in the form of mutual assistance, spotting and securing, for cooperative, interactive, communicative and problem-solving behavior
- Cooperation means practicing in small groups, which promotes self-reliance and responsibility

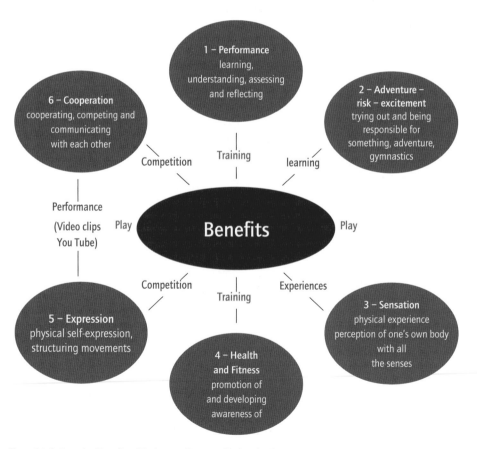

Figure 14: Pedagogical benefits of Parkour and Freerunning in schools

7.2   CONTENTS AND ACTIVITIES

PARKOUR IS RUNNING AND JUMPING!

From a pupil's perspective, the movements have **structural similarities**, especially with **gymnastics** movements, which cannot be disputed by the Parkour scene. Alongside the gymnastic-type basic forms of supporting, hanging, balancing and rolling, there are also gymnastic skills that are reflected in Parkour and Freerunning movements. The basic elements of Parkour that have emerged in recent years simply have a lot in common with gymnastic elements, they have just been given different names. For example, a clearance that in Parkour is called a Kong or a Monkey is called a tuck vault in gymnastics.

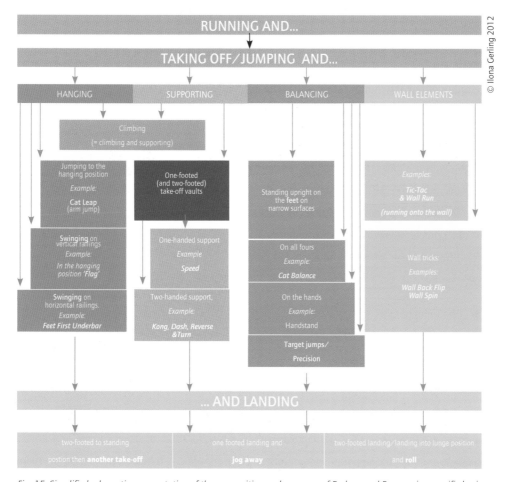

© Ilona Gerling 2012

Fig. 15: Simplified schematic representation of the composition and sequence of Parkour and Freerunning-specific basic movement forms and basic skills (basic elements).

Parkour is running, taking off and landing. Before the landing, the type of situation or environment requires a certain type of movement solution. This can be a support or a hang; it can be the way the movement is structured. Climbing and balancing challenges can also be added to the above basic movement forms to allow the individual, probably also the more efficient way to be sought. With this basic model in mind, the teacher can also build obstacles with gymnastics apparatus to elicit a variety of movements (see figure 15).

A teacher teaching Parkour is at an advantage if he has a good knowledge of gymnastics. Parkour also contains elements of track and field: running fast, long and high jumping. These foundations allow tips to be given for implementing movement solutions in movement tasks, and also, based on an understanding of these movement forms, make a sense of achievement possible even in the short time available for school classes via methodical introductions.

7.3 BASIC PRINCIPLES OF CURRICULUM STRUCTURE

Pupil-oriented: individualization and inclusion

In order to cater for the different prerequisites, interests and abilities of the children.

Individualization through differentiation

Along with the *movement tasks*, the (above mentioned) structures, apparatus and equipment layouts determine the movements produced!

The stimulus of specific obstacles produces the movement result.

In schools, always select the apparatus obstacle that triggers the set movement task for different levels of ability. In short, **all** pupils must be able to perform the Parkour tasks, whether by

- Changing heights
- Changing distances of the apparatus
- Using auxiliary equipment
- Varying the amount of partner assistance given

This offers opportunities to reflect on individual limits, adventure and risk, and security. Especially during the pupils' self-active work, the teacher must observe, control and advise them to monitor the apparatus structures and the movement solutions performed on them from a security perspective, and if necessary even to ask them not to do certain things, as he bears the ultimate responsibility for their safety.

Provide subject-specific foundations and promote active, autonomous, cooperative work: open and guided/free and compulsory

More than ever, schools are insisting that pupils perceive, experience and learn from a range of experiences, experiments, mistakes, structures and risk in their actions. This type of learning addresses other regions of the brain than does purely learning by rote. It has been proven that the retention of acquired knowledge is significantly enhanced by actively engaging with the learning object (e.g., by self-active work in small groups).

Individual movement solutions are only achieved via open tasks and thus by individual learning phases. One of the definitions of Parkour is the finding of individual/original movements! Finding one's own movement possibilities with results where the aim is (here in the truest sense of the word) overcoming obstacles requires that time for movement

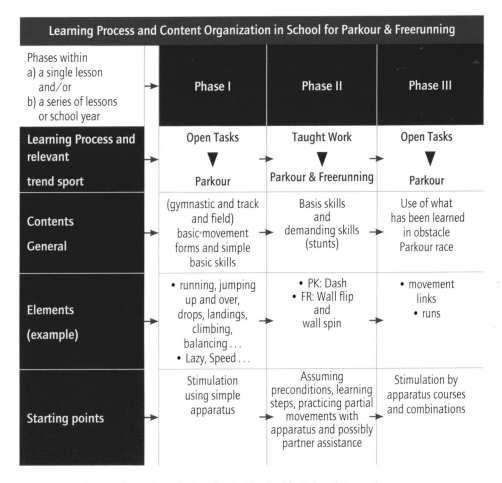

Learning Process and Content Organization in School for Parkour & Freerunning			
Phases within a) a single lesson and/or b) a series of lessons or school year	Phase I	Phase II	Phase III
Learning Process and relevant trend sport	Open Tasks ▼ Parkour	Taught Work ▼ Parkour & Freerunning	Open Tasks ▼ Parkour
Contents General	(gymnastic and track and field) basic movement forms and simple basic skills	Basis skills and demanding skills (stunts)	Use of what has been learned in obstacle Parkour race
Elements (example)	• running, jumping up and over, drops, landings, climbing, balancing … • Lazy, Speed …	• PK: Dash • FR: Wall flip and wall spin	• movement links • runs
Starting points	Stimulation using simple apparatus	Assuming preconditions, learning steps, practicing partial movements with apparatus and possibly partner assistance	Stimulation by apparatus courses and combinations

Figure 16: Learning procedure and organization of content in school for Parkour & Freerunning

experimentation is provided so that each pupil can learn in his own time and by developing his own learning strategies.

Reduced school hours and the inadequate conditioning and coordinative prerequisites of the pupils represent problems for the schools. If the basic movement forms of running, jumping, climbing and balancing are to be mastered on appropriate apparatus by every pupil and in open movement tasks in the initial, warm-up phase of the Parkour class and series of classes (see figure 16), then many pupils will already have reached their limits even before being introduced to the first Parkour skills.

The teacher is also responsible for the tasks he sets his pupils. In a series of six physical education classes, though he must ultimately draw on his knowledge, experience progress and step-by-step learning in order to enable all pupils to experience a sense of achievement. Cumulative learning is used as the foundation for open task setting in the higher levels that follow and also to protect the pupils from injury.

To summarize: the ideal lesson format is the "sandwich model," where phases of teaching, collective learning and open "individual" learning alternate.

Freedom is a term that is mentioned again and again by Parkour supporters. There is nothing you are not allowed to do; there is no right or wrong. Nobody tells you what to do or how to do it. You try things out, exchange tips with others and find your own way.

Independent, self-active and movement-creative work on open tasks is one of the goals of a good physical education class. Exactly this can be achieved with Parkour. Such a class is much more difficult than a "taught class," as it requires significantly more expert knowledge and experience of movement situations.

CLASS GOALS: IMPLEMENTATION AND TRANSFER/PRACTICING AND IMPLEMENTATION
... in order to acquire sufficient confidence in the newly acquired movement repertoire. What has been learned must be put into practice and class situations must be created in which what has been learned can be implemented and presented. Skills development leads to improved self-esteem and more successes. The motivation to keep on practicing also grows. In Parkour, successful stunts are performed in front of others. At the end of the class and/or a series of classes, the goal will always be to incorporate new skills into the obstacle course runs, which also involves self-evaluation, evaluation by others and performance.

LEARNING AND UNDERSTANDING

Students should strive to gain awareness of the practical doing and learning, in order to incorporate this successfully into the next practical action. Pupils must be given space to reflect or what has been learned must be discussed.

Problem-oriented teaching and opening up interlinking interdisciplinary learning chances

The goal is to use the acquired skills in an inter-disciplinary way and bring them into other areas of life. Links to other disciplines and school subjects should be exploited. Pupils can, for example, at the start of a series of classes acquire rudimentary Parkour skills by being set the task of researching different Parkour techniques for clearing obstacles on the Internet. At the end of a series of classes, a video clip can be produced in a school video club using footage filmed in Parkour classes. Complex tasks should also be set that are geared to implementation and transfer as well.

© Michael Schaab

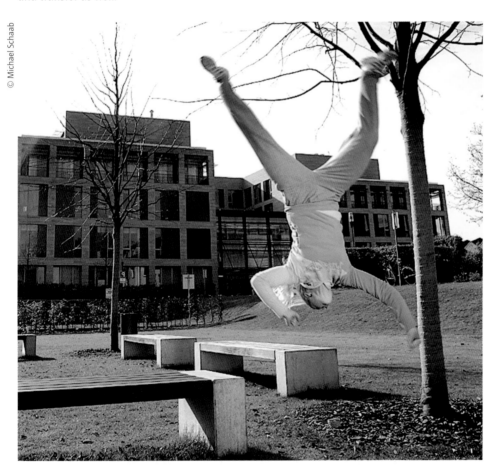

7.4   SAFETY

To avoid Parkour and Freerunning-related accidents, the following guidelines should be observed in schools.

Basic conditions for security

Professional competence and methodical approach

■ The teachers should possess **knowledge of the theoretical foundation of the basic techniques** of track and field and gymnastics, and have acquired knowledge of the specific basic movement forms in Parkour and Freerunning.

■ The tasks set for pupils must correspond to their **abilities and social maturity**.

■ All tasks must be able to demonstrate **a methodical approach**, in the event of an accident.

■ Teachers must master **spotting and securing** and be able to teach pupils how to do this step by step. However, teachers should be prepared to spot and secure themselves on demanding activity stations.

Landing and falling protection

■ Drops from heights **above** reachable height must not be allowed without appropriate landing mats in order to avoid landings that overload the joints.

■ Particular attention should be paid to healthy, technically proficient landing techniques. These must be practiced adequately under simplified conditions before being performed from greater heights or under time pressure as part of movement combinations.

■ Suitable **fall protection** (mats) must be provided. Use as many mats as necessary or as few as possible so that pupils don't land on mat edges when running and jumping, and also to simulate outdoor conditions. Both over and under-protection should be avoided.

■ **Appropriate landing surfaces** for the level of mastery of the movements and the heights of the obstacles should be chosen. The gym floor is sufficient for running up to, from and over simple obstacles, as well as for balancing movements on beams below hip-height. Gymnastics mats or large landing mats should be placed behind boxes above hip-height. Thick mats should be placed behind horizontal bars that are to be cleared, where there is a danger of pupils falling on their heads. The same is true for wall bars from which drops are performed from a great height. As well as the complexity of a movement, it is ultimately the height of the drop that determines the choice of mat protection. Remember, for Parkour, use as many mats as necessary and as few mats as possible.

Apparatus and first aid box

- **The apparatus** must be tested for resilience and stability and set up to suit the movements. Small block boxes that are to be jumped onto must for example be placed horizontally (grip hole facing the approaching pupil) so that they don't tip over.
- First aid box must be available.

  Where is it? Does it contain the necessary items? Must it be opened with a key? Where is the key? Who may have it? Is the emergency phone number at hand?

Methodical To-Dos

- **Create prerequisites and work step by step!**
- Always start training/practice with a **warm-up** to stimulate circulation and blood supply to the muscles, but also use tasks and warm-up games to stimulate reaction ability, alertness and attention levels.
- **Start with simple exercise forms** and constantly work on the basic movement forms, repeating them in every class until they are mastered, especially before they are implemented on outdoors terrain. Include already learned and mastered movements (stunts) in the introductory section.
- Always start working at ground level with **mats, spotters and aids** (auxiliary equipment).
- The **spotters** must be clear about the **responsibility** they have toward their fellow pupils. Spotting grips must be demonstrated, explained and tried out in simple situations.
- The pupils must, if they are over-enthusiastic, be told not to try to do too much and not to **try to implement demanding elements too soon**. The body needs time to adapt to the demands.
- The pupils must be told that they must be careful and vigilant at all times.

SET RULES AND HAVE THE PUPILS ACCEPT THEM

RULES FOR TRACEURS AND FREERUNNERS

- *Always use your head first before giving free rein to your emotions or moving a muscle.*
- *Always make sure that the "move" is safe.*
- *Do not rush or make unpremeditated moves.*
- *Never overestimate your ability.*
- *Never practice demanding elements alone.*
- *Never practice alone in an unsafe and unfamiliar area. Someone must always be present in case of emergency.*
- *Every obstacle must be taken seriously, even if you have already overcome it many times before.*
- *No pressure! Nobody HAS TO do anything!*
- *No traceur or freerunner should be compelled, incited or forced by the group to do something in order to prove himself.*
- *Parkour and freerunning are "art forms based on movement and the creative invention of tricks," which are intended to train mind and body. Dares and showing off are taboo on the scene!*

RULES FOR OUTDOORS

It is a big step to take a school group from the gym to the outdoor terrain. This is the ultimate goal for young people who are familiar with the movements, the feeling and scene from Internet videos on YouTube. Only outdoors can a student of Parkour become a traceur.

What should the person responsible for taking his pupils outdoors bear in mind?

OUTDOOR RULES

- All participants will be **part of the environment used**. As a part of the environment, one must adapt to it. That means, for example, that the **environment must be respected** and it must be treated with respect. Likewise, private property as well as public spaces must not be abused. Traceurs do not alter their obstacles, they look for those that are appropriate for their movements and constantly adapt their movements to the characteristics of each new obstacle.
- **Movements** must **be adequately prepared indoors**, possibly with the help of partners, aids and mats for security, before being put into practice outdoors. This can apply to the conditioning-coordination prerequisites, as well as the skill levels of the basic elements of PK.

- Teachers teaching outdoors must **have acquired prior practical experience of the elements indoors**, not only in order to be able to give valuable tips to ensure quick results but above all so that they can very quickly **spot moments of danger** during transfer situations and be able to intervene rapidly and appropriately.

- Teachers must have checked the outdoor **obstacle and landing areas** thoroughly and conscientiously before they are used by the pupils. Landing areas must be examined (stones removed, for example), soft surfaces and sandy ground (e.g., in playgrounds) are preferable for landings from great heights.

- Outdoors too, teachers must prepare the pupils adequately physically, co-ordinatively and mentally **for the challenges to follow**. This includes slow warm-up runs, reaction activities, games of tag, as well as stationary stretching exercises.

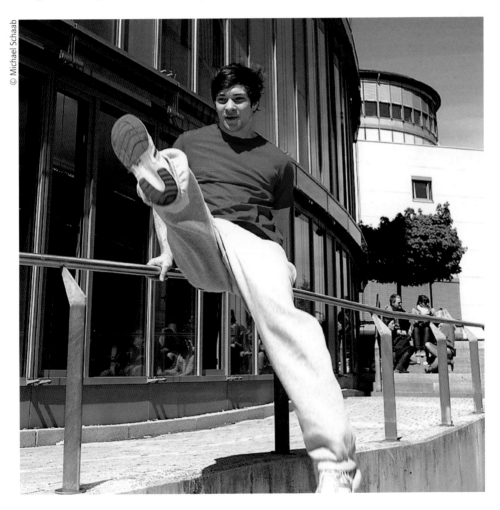

© Michael Schaab

7.5   LESSON PLANS

7.5.1   BASIC STRUCTURES

The lesson plans are structured with the intention to be conducted during block schedules.

- In order to have enough time for finding, structuring, rejecting, changing and performing movement solutions.
- So that it is worthwhile putting out extensive amounts of apparatus and to be able to rearrange, combine and rearrange them again. The ratio of effort to benefit must be reasonable, which ultimately depends on the amount of time available.

The gym must be large enough to allow

- small groups to work well side by side
- for runs over the obstacles so that a flow can be experienced
- enough room for a lot of apparatus, including fixed apparatus

The double period must be well-structured.

- Introduction:
    - Presentation of class content and goals
    - Explain terminology
    - Collect pupils' homework
    - Video contributions
    - Music suggestions

- Practical Introduction: running work with theme-specific additional activities
    - Awakening attention and reaction ability
    - Stimulation of the cardiovascular system
    - Preparation of the muscles by running and gentle stretching
    - Link together simple theme-specific movement forms (e.g. landing and supporting)
    - Obstacle races over simple obstacles
    - Possibly repeating and consolidating Parkour movements from previous lessons

- Emphasis
    - To be worked on open activities or taught activities.

- **Final Phase**
  - Perform/present/compare/play
  - Cool down
- **End of the lesson plan**
  - Reflecting, offering possibility of discussion, getting feedback
  - Summarizing content and goals
  - Possibly giving homework
  - Looking ahead at the next class (possibly structured with pupil's help)

7.5.2   SIX SIMPLIFIED EXAMPLE LESSON PLANS

The content of these six lesson plans was chosen to give pupils basic knowledge of the trend sports Parkour and Freerunning.

1st Lesson Plan

Topic – **Parkour running**, overcoming obstacles
Main pedagogical aim: promoting health, developing awareness of health
Other pedagogical aims:
- Improving sensory perception, extending movement experience and physical experience
- Cooperating, competing and communicating

Contents of the lesson plan	Intentions
• Gathering pupils' existing knowledge of Parkour • Watching a video clip example and identifying features of Parkour • Set homework at the end of class with the pupils **Aim:** Google Parkour on the Internet	• Introduction to the series of Parkour classes • Establishing which pupils are already experts • If necessary, picking "pupil experts" for the groups to be formed
Running and clearing obstacles	• Gaining initial, simple Parkour experiences • Learning to evaluate one's own movement abilities and skills
Running and working out individual and varied clearance techniques	• Finding movement solutions • Working out individualmovement possibilities
Changing the height of and distance between obstacles	Teams cooperate in changing their Parkour course
Independent and criteria-led building of an obstacle running course	Teams communicate and exchange obstacles for other apparatus and combinations
Fast and sustained running	• Stimulation of the cardiovascular system and experiencing improvement of (speed) strength, endurance flow as flying
Fast obstacle running in comparison	Implementation of movement under time pressure and in competition

EXAMPLE OF A LAYOUT

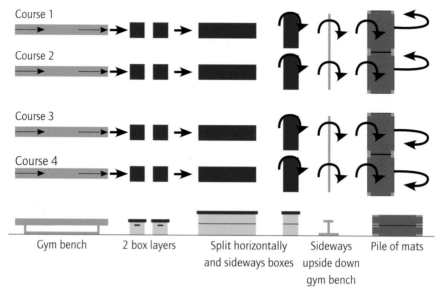

| Gym bench | 2 box layers | Split horizontally and sideways boxes | Sideways upside down gym bench | Pile of mats |

SUGGESTIONS FOR RUNNING COURSES

- Obstacle course can be run over, then pupils run their own path back to the start
- Obstacle courses can be run in both directions
- First course down, second course back, third course down again and fourth course back to start at the narrow end of the sports hall again
- Courses 1 and 4 and courses 2 and 3 can be run in a circuit

At the end of a course, in the last third of the class, box steps can also be set up that must be run up. A special incentive can be given for those who jump up from the box steps to hang on the high bar or from the top bar of the uneven bars.

Fit pupils can even jump onto the wall bars (apparatus layout, see figure 17)

Tip: Place feet first onto the wall bars or the mats leaning on them, then grip the top bar in a crouched hang.

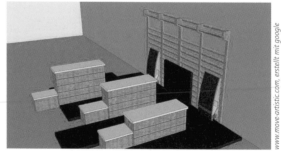

www.move-artistic.com, erstellt mit google

sketch up

Figure 17: Run up a pile of boxes and jump up to hang from the knees from the wall bars.

© Michael Schaab

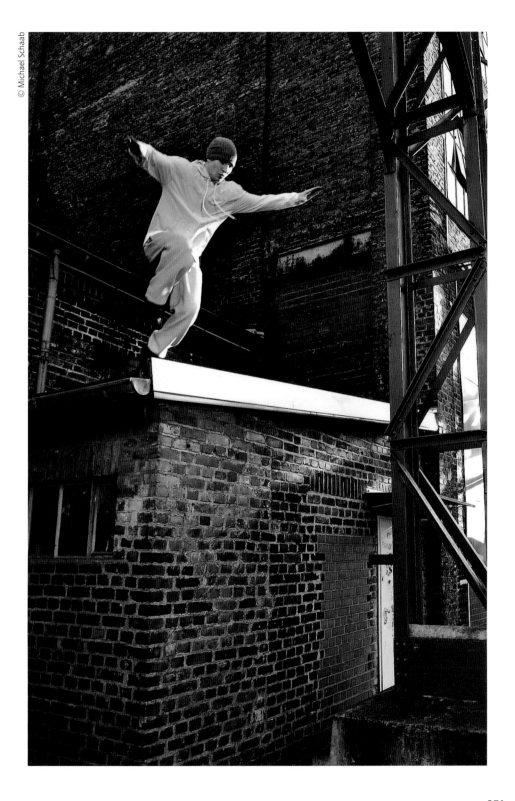

2nd Lesson Plan

Topic – Parkour running, Vaulting, overcoming obstacles: familiarization with vaults/clearance techniques

Main pedagogical aim: cooperation, competition and communication
Other pedagogical aims: taking risks and responsibility. Physical self-expression, structuring movement.

Contents of the lesson plan	Intentions
• Collect results of homework "Parkour on the Internet," show and analyze a selection. • Set new homework: look for running music for the end of the coming class	• Familiarization with Parkour vaults from the scene • Involvement of the pupils in the lesson plan and adaptation to needs of young people
Running and clearing higher obstacles that make a vault necessary	Learning to evaluate one's own movement abilities and skills.
• Familiarization with supporting Parkour moves, running and working out individual and complex support-jump-clearance techniques • Examples: from leg tuck to Kong, from crouch jump to reverse, from supported scissor jump and/or from running Kehre to Speed, etc.	• Finding movement solutions, working out individual movement possibilities • Producing one's own "special physical performance" (Crick, 2008) • Learning the process of working out a movement solution
Changing the obstacles	Teams cooperate in changing their obstacle course
Independent and criteria-led building of an obstacle vaulting course	Teams communicate and exchange obstacles for other apparatus and combinations
• Fast and sustained vaulting over obstacles	Stimulation of the cardiovascular system and experiencing improvement of (speed) strength, endurance flow as flying

APPARATUS STRUCTURES

Examples of apparatus structures for running and vaulting over obstacles can be found in Chapter 4.5 "Vaults."

3rd Lesson Plan

Topic – **Parkour** running, supporting, balancing and climbing, overcoming obstacles

Main pedagogical aim: physical self-expression, structuring movement
Other pedagogical aims: taking risks and responsibility

Contents of the lesson plan	Intentions
Running and balancing	Learning to evaluate one's own movement abilities and skills
Running and working out individual and varied clearances of different kinds of obstacles	Finding movement solutions, working out individual movement possibilities
Changing the obstacles and combinations of obstacles	Teams cooperate in changing their Parkour course
Independent and criteria-led construction of a varied Parkour course	Teams communicate with each other and exchange obstacles with other apparatus and combinations
Presentation of an individually worked out Parkour sequence as an individual run and in groups to self-selected music	• Implementation of the movement, demonstration of movement ideas and a flowing running link in Parkour • Learning a feeling of flow and aesthetic movement experience as a movement motivation

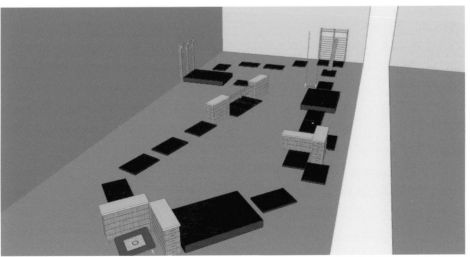

www.move-artistic.com, erstellt mit google sketch up

Figure 18: Jumping, vaulting, climbing and balancing circuit

Ask more able pupils to climb up an apparatus combination in the middle or at the end of the obstacle course (figure 18) formed of horizontal uneven bars (remove one bar) and high steps formed of boxes. The box steps are to be approached from all sides. Approach from the bar side, and use the bar to grip with the hands, as they would for a cat leap/arm jump (the feet support the lift onto the box. The horizontal box behind the high sideways box also serves to stabilize the high box!).

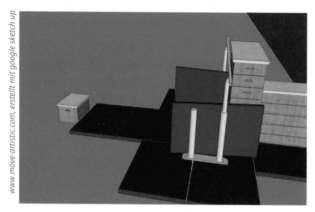

www.move-artistic.com, erstellt mit google sketch up

Figure 19: Apparatus layout bar and box combination for running up, vaulting, hanging and final dismount.

A versatile apparatus layout can be created if the apparatus are arranged more compactly and centrally. With boxes, small box blocks/sections and gym benches, which are part of the basic equipment of any gym, you can build box lanes, raised balancing courses and areas for running jumps/precision landings from several sides (figure 19).

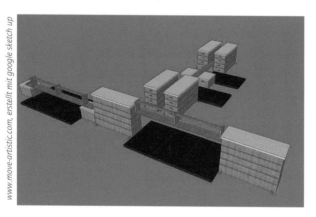

www.move-artistic.com, erstellt mit google sketch up

Figure 20: Apparatus arrangement for climbing, vaulting, balancing and precision landing.

4th Lesson Plan

Topic – Parkour learning **Parkour techniques: Dash Vault and feet first underbar.**

Main pedagogical aim: taking risks and learning responsibility
Other pedagogical aims: learning, understanding and evaluating performances

Contents of the lesson plan	Intentions
Running and clearing obstacles feet first, supporting the clearance by hanging and supporting	• Learning unusual, tricky and new types of movements • Daring to jump feet first over an obstacle and only then using the hands • Taking responsibility for which learning steps can be mastered and which heights can be attempted
• Learning and practicing two basic Parkour techniques: Dash and Feet First Underbar	• Autonomous practicing in groups at stations • Teams cooperate at their stations
• Using learning facilities and supporting others as they learn movements	• Correcting, helping and encouraging them
• Stations 1 and 2: one-footed take-off from sitting position on a hip-high pile of soft mats • Station 1: see above with box placed in front, support on the box as preparation for the Dash Vault • Station 2: see above with grip on an overhead horizontal bar as preparation for the Feet First Underbar • Station 3: Dash over low box (lay a pile of mats as a landing mat, 1-2 spotters secure the pupils' backs to keep them from falling backwards) • Station 4: Feet First Underbar at the horizontal bar over obstacles (pile of mats for landing mat. The height is initially provided by an elastic rope/rope then by box sections or gym benches and finally by large boxes or a hip-high second horizontal bar (see page 206)	• Experiencing potential risk as a positive thing • Experiencing success in terms of enjoyment and movement motivation • Overcoming fear • Trying out the unknown • Undertaking movement experiments
Parkour as the presentation of what has been learned: demonstration of the Dash and Underbar techniques in a flowing Parkour running combination	• Use of the movement • Being aware of skills • Improving self-awareness, self-esteem and self-confidence

TIP:

A box "lane" (figure 21) can be constructed for trying out the Dash Vault for the return run as the third station. If another rope is placed above the boxes at the end of the box lane for added difficulty, the feet must be raised clearly over the height of the boxes. A springboard or a small horizontally box section can be used as a take-off aid. The landing area should be sufficiently covered in landing mats and then removed when the pupils have gained more confidence.

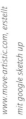

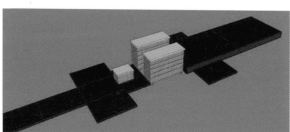

Figure 21: Box "lane" for practicing

the Dash Vault

5th Lesson Plan

Topic – Parkour – learning a) **Tic-Tac** running technique onto a wall
b) **Freerunning technique: Wall back flip**
c) Learn **to help each other**

Main pedagogical aim: improving perception, extending movement experience
Other pedagogical aims: a) Learning, understanding and evaluating performances
b) Cooperation and communication

Contents of the lesson plan	Intentions
Learning to run onto the wall (Tic-Tac)	Daring to run up the wall on the feet
• Learning a flip movement on the wall • Learning and consolidating technical skills • Identifying structures of movement technique	• Learning unusual, tricky and new types of movements • Daring to jump head over heels and backward • Experiencing potential risk as a positive thing • Experiencing success in terms of enjoyment and movement motivation • Overcoming fear • Trying out the unknown • Engaging in movement experiments

- Familiarity with and use of security measures and spotters
- Developing trust in spotters and security measures

- Autonomous practice in groups at stations
- Teams cooperate, correct, help and encourage each other
- Taking responsibility when spotting
- Responsibility for oneself as to what and how much help one needs

Parkour as a presentation of what has been learned	• Implementation of movement • Demonstration of wall back flip • Improving self-esteem and self-confidence

6th Lesson Plan

Topic – Parkour   a) **Constructing** a Parkour run to film
b) **Presentation and recording of** a worked-out Parkour sequence as group effort performance

Main pedagogical aim: learning, understanding and evaluating performance
Other pedagogical aims: cooperation and communication

Contents of the lesson plan	Intentions
Constructing a small Parkour course in groups	• Teams cooperate
Planning a video recording	• Organizing a video recording; establishing a direction plan
Warming up	• Planning and execution of special Parkour warm-up exercises
Practicing the selected elements	• Team members help each other
Practicing links	• Team members interact, agree, solve problems, support each other.
• Knowing and implementing organizational criteria • Cooperating and communicating with others • Parkour as presentation of what has been learned • Creating a video recording	• Being aware of skills, improving self-confidence and self-esteem • Documentation of individual and group performances of a learning process over six classes in the presentation • Learning how to set criteria for individual performance and group organization • Implementation of the movement products, demonstration of the learned Parkour and Freerunning techniques in a flowing Parkour run • Presentation of the result

The possibilities for setting up Parkour structures are endless. In each small group, the solutions for tackling the set task will be different, depending on the skill, interest, number and type of available apparatus and depending on the creativity of the pupils. One example layout is presented to inspire you (figures 22a/b).

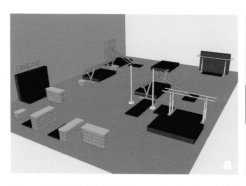 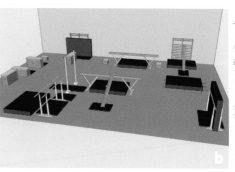

www.move-artistic.com, erstellt mit google sketch up

Figures 22a/b: Varied obstacle course for clearing and balancing in the sports hall (seen from two perspectives)

CONCLUSION

And at the end of the school year, the video production is watched and celebrated together in a party. It will certainly not take long for it to end up on YouTube. Who will receive the most views, the highest ratings and comments? That can also be celebrated at the end of the school year with the election of a winning group J!

Have fun and good luck!

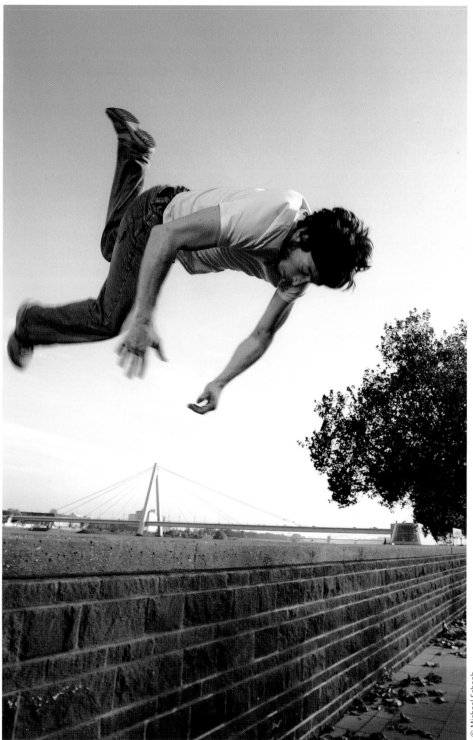

© Michael Schaab

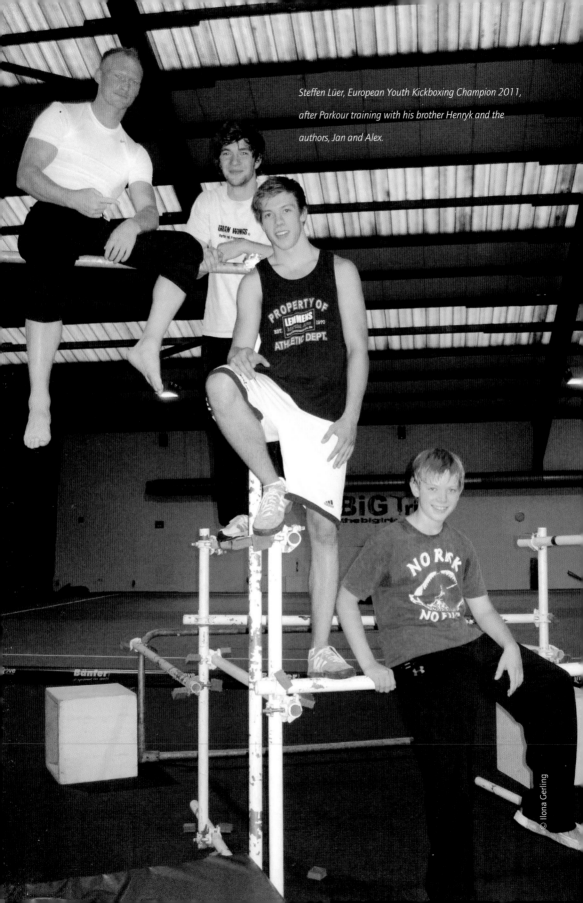

Steffen Lüer, European Youth Kickboxing Champion 2011, after Parkour training with his brother Henryk and the authors, Jan and Alex.

© Ilona Cerling

8   THE PK/FR LEXICON

8.1 STANDING   POSITIONS RELATIVE TO THE OBSTACLE

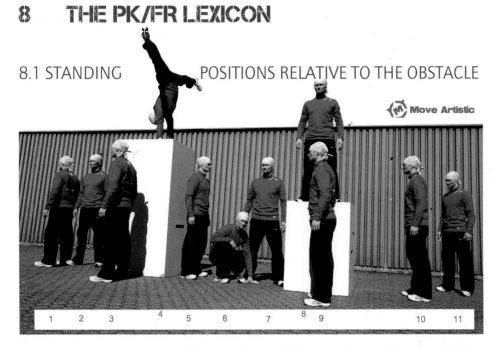

If the obstacle is simple (e.g., block, box or rail), the following standing positions are possible:

- Relative to side of the body: **facing toward – facing away from – diagonally**
- Relative to the body's lateral axis: **parallel – cross – diagonal**

For two imaginary longitudinal axes parallel to the ground, by both obstacles, the positions, whether one stands between or outside the obstacles, have additional terms **inside or outside** (as with bars).

The traceur can stand as follows:

Position 1	(outside) parallel (facing away)
Position 2	(outside) crossways (sideways on)
Position 3	(outside) parallel
Position 4	(parallel) handstand on the obstacle
Position 5	(inside) parallel
Position 6	(inside) parallel crouched
Position 7	(inside) crossways
Position 8	sideways on the obstacle
Position 9	(outside) parallel (sideways)
Position 10	(outside) diagonal (facing toward)
Position 11	(outside) diagonal (facing forward)
Position 12	(outside) crossways (facing forward)

8.2 AXES OF ROTATION

Parkour and Freerunning moves are three-dimensional movements in space. Traceurs and freerunners turn through different body axes when performing original movements. The greater the number of rotations and the more different axes that the rotations pass though, the more spectacular the moves. There are three main axes through which the body rotates (see photo).

A   LONGITUDINAL AXIS

Example: twist and spiral Underbar

B   TRANSVERSAL AXIS

Example: Front Flip, Wall Flip, Feet First Underbar, Dash and Kong

C   SAGITTAL AXIS

Example: Side Flip and Aerial

D   BENT AXIS

Example: Parkour Roll

As mentioned above, these are the main axes. The most original moves turn through all possible combinations of these axes.

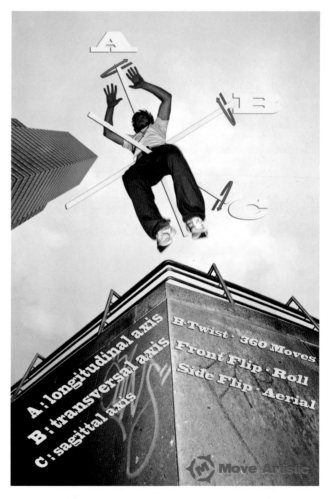

Axes of Rotation

8.3 SUPPORT AND HANG GRIPS

Different support and hang grips are used in Parkour and Freerunning to clear and cross obstacles. The grips used are grouped into categories below.

8.3.1 SUPPORT GRIPS

Overhand Grip

The backs of the Hands face upward or forward, the thumbs point towards each other

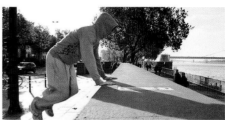

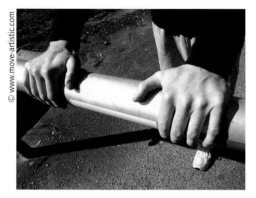

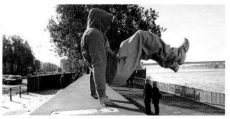

Example: Kash

Spokebone Grip

The palms of the hands face each other and the thumbs point forward

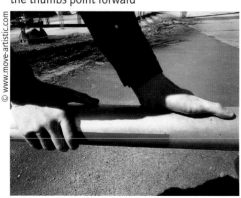

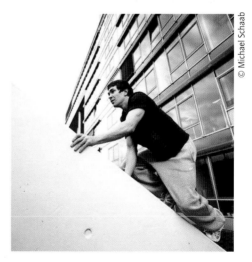

Example: Cat Balance

Ulnagrip

One hand grips overhand and the other underhand grips so that the heels of the hands point outward.

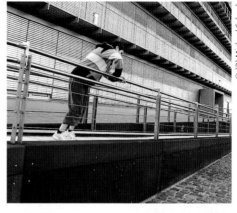

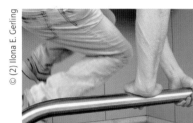

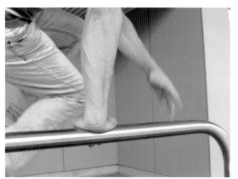

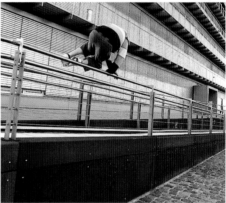

Example: Reverse

Mixed Grip

The mixed grip is a combination of overhand and underhand grip

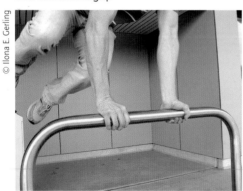

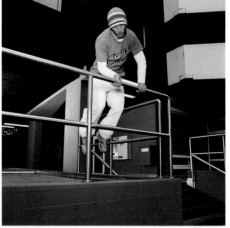

Example: Turn

Mixed Support Grips

Simple supports and support with grip on the edge

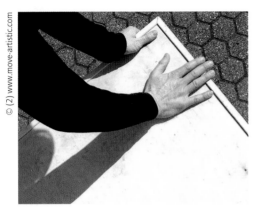 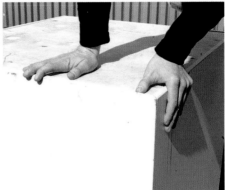

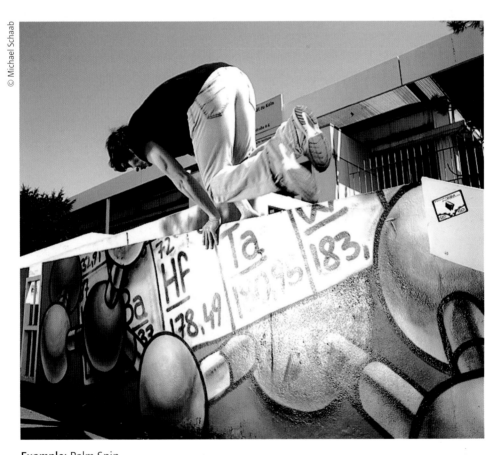

Example: Palm Spin

8.3.2   HANG GRIPS

Overhand Grip

The backs of the hands face back or down, the thumbs face each other (also in the Monkey Grip, see photo with overhand grip on the edge)

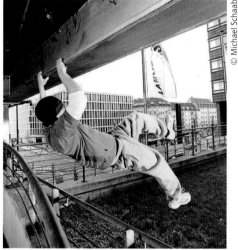

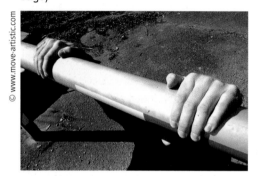

Example: Feet First Underbar

Underhand Grip

The backs of the hands face forward, the thumbs point outward

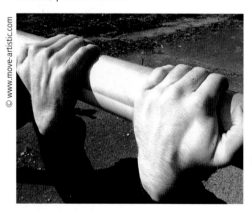

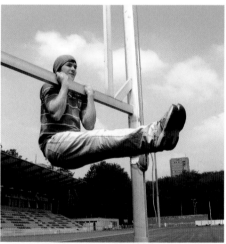

Example: pull-up

Mixed Grip

The mixed grip is a combination of the overhand and underhand grips

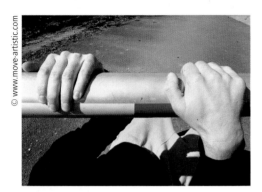

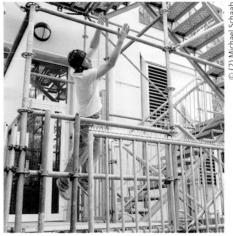

Example: Spiral Underbar

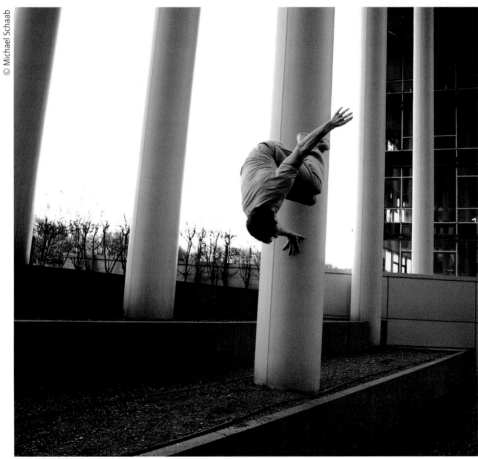

8.4   GLOSSARY OF PARKOUR AND FREERUNNING TECHNIQUES

The majority of the techniques described below have already been covered in detail in the movement descriptions earlier in this book. However, they are also listed below in concise form in English and French.

English	French
Balance (4,5)	Équilibre (5)
Cat Balance (4)	
Handstand (4)	
Flag (4)	
Cat Walking (3)	Quadrupédie (3)
Standing Jump/s (3/5)	Saut à l'arrêt (3)
Running Jumps (5)	Saut de détente (1,2)/ Saut d'élan (2)
Drop Jumps (5)/ Dismount (4)/ Forward/Drop (5)	Saut de fond (1,2)
Precision (3)	Saut de précision (1,2,3)
Standing Precision Jump (5)	
Precision – 1-foot (4)	
Precision – 2-foot (4)	
Running Precision (4)	

Explanation

Balancing means keeping one's body
in equilibrium against the forces of gravity

Balance on all fours on narrow surfaces (e.g., on a rail)

Balancing with an extended body on the hands

Power balance with the hands gripping a vertical pole, with the arms,
upper body and ideally also the legs in a horizontal position

Moving forward on the hands and feet (crawling)

Jump from standing without an approach

Running jump with one-footed take-off
for distance or over a certain distance then jog or roll away

Depth jump from high level to floor

Jumps with precision landing onto limited landing area

Precision jumps from standing (without approach)

One-footed take-off

Two-footed take-off, one-footed landing

Precision jumps with approach

English	French
Tic-Tac (3,6)/ Tic-Tac (4)/ (Stepping Movements (5))	Tic-tac (1,5,6)/tic-tac (2,3)
Tic Tac 180°	
Tic Tac 360° (5)	
Tic Tac to Crane (4)	
Tic Tac to Precision (4)	
Tic Tac to Cat (4)	
Vaults (5)	Passe barrière (2)/ passement (1,2,3,5)
	Demi-tour (6)
Step Vault (5)	Passement rapide (6)
Lazy Vault (3,4)	Passement latéral
Lazy to Drop	
Lazy Gainer (Source: YouTube: Lazygainer – Brand New Move January 2008)	
Lateral Vault (5)	

Explanation

Approach and push-off from the wall or similar vertical surface to
one-footed push-off as redirection of the movement direction or
as push-off aid to hang or before clearing an obstacle

Both feet are placed on the wall with simultaneous body rotation around
the longitudinal axis. The foot that is placed second on the wall is used as a fast ,powerful
push-off. The hands can also be used to push off from the wall.

Tic-Tac with complete rotation

Tic-Tac to one-footed Crane landing

Tic-Tac with precision landing

Tic-Tac followed by Cat Leap

Different clearance techniques with the assistance of the supporting hands.
A vault is the term used for supported jumps, *passement* is understood
by Parkour aficionados as the general term for clearance techniques. Usually, one-footed
running take-off then one-footed landing and jog away.

Take-off to support (on railing to mixed grip)
and a half turn jump over the obstacle to land parallel,
the front is facing the obstacle throughout.

Vault in which the body goes sideways/facing away from the obstacle,
the near take-off leg is tucked up close to the body during clearance and brought forward to
land (take-off leg = landing leg) without touching the obstacle.
The free leg is above the tucked up leg.

A supported scissors jump with the back turned to the apparatus,
one-footed take-off and one-footed landing then jog away.
The *passement latéral* is executed from a parallel run to the obstacle (6)

Lazy from a great height. Close the legs and two-handed guidance
and/or two-handed push-off in the desired direction of landing

After a Lazy, a back flip at right-angles to the initial direction of movement
is added in before landing

Sideways jumping technique with different possible executions,
the side of the body faces the apparatus during the supported clearance

English	French
Vaults (5)	**Passe barrière (2)/ passement (1,2,3,5)**
Kong Vault (4,5)/ Cat Path (3)/Monkey (5)	Saut de chat (1,2,5)/ passement de chat (3)
Diving Kong (4)	
Kong to Precision (4)	
Kong to Cat (Leap)	
Double Kong (4)	
Triple Kong	
Kong 360° (Source: YouTube: Paul, R "360°– Kong Vault")	
Speed Vault (3,4)	Passement speed (3)
Dash Vault (3,4)	Passement assis (3)
Dash Bomb (YouTube: "Ronnie Shalvis Dash Bomb!" (Landed Outside))	
Kash Vault (4)	
Reverse (3)/ Reverse Vault (4)	Réverse (1)/ passement arrière (3)
Reverse to Cat	
Turn Vault (4,5)	Demi-tour (1,2)

Explanation

Different clearance techniques with the assistance of the supporting hands.
A vault is the term used for supported jumps, *passement* is understood
by Parkour aficionados as the general term for clearance techniques.
Take-offs are usually one-footed running and landings are one-footed into a jog.

Kong Vault from approach and with one-footed
or two-footed take-off to one-footed landing and jog away

Long first flight phase before the support phase when performing
a tuck vault over an obstacle

Kong Vault to precision

Kong Vault followed by Arm Jump/Cat Leap

Kong Vault with double support when performing tuck vault over an obstacle

Kong Vault with triple support when performing a tuck vault over an obstacle

Complete rotation before and in the first flight phase into a Kong Vault
followed immediately by supported tuck vault over an obstacle

Sideways stance to the obstacle to be cleared with one-handed
support during the push-off phase

A feet-first jump in which the legs cross the obstacle supported by the hands

Dash Vault with push-off and from a supported position,
before the landing, push-off into forward flip

Combination of Kong Vault and Dash Vault (double hand support phase)

360° rotation over the obstacle, crossing it with one's back to it

Supported vault facing the obstacle followed by rotation around the longitudinal axis with
the back to the obstacle followed by landing in the Cat Leap position

Jump with change of obstacle side, after landing
parallel stand facing and in front of the obstacle

English	French
Vaults (5)	Passe barrière (2)/ passement (1,2,3,5)
Palm Spin (4)	
Palm Spin 360°	
Landing (3)/ Landing basics (5)	Réception (2,3)
Drops	
Dismounts	Saut de fond
Straight Landing (5)	
Staggered Landing (5)	
Crane (4)/Crane Jump (5)	
Crane Moon Step (4)	
Landing from a Drop (4)	

Explanation

Different clearance techniques with the assistance of the supporting hands.
A vault is the term used for supported jumps, *passement* is understood
by Parkour aficionados as the general term for clearance techniques. Usually,
take-offs are one-footed running and landings one-footed then jog away.

Rotation around one hand (palm of the hand) on an obstacle,
so that the take-off side is also the landing side

Palm Spin with landing facing the obstacle in order to take it again

Landing

(Passive) dropping from heights with active landing on the feet

Active jumping down landing on the feet

Straight landing on the same level as the take-off

Landing on limited landing area, where the landing is unlike the take-off angle
and the feet land one after the other (e.g., jump with a quarter turn and landing
on a narrow ledge or wall)

The Crane or Crane Landing is a one-footed landing with a bent landing knee
on the obstacle and support of the hanging foot,
which acts as it does in the arm jump (with the ball of the foot)
in order to stop the forward momentum

Special form of Wall Run with push-off to Crane Landing,
in order to arrive directly on the obstacle with one foot
so that the take-off foot is also the landing foot.
The knee of the free leg is pulled up
and the take-off foot follows it to land.
To the observer, this looks like a step in the air, or a Moon Step.
This technique became famous due to the technique videos of Urban Freeflow.
In the video, the traceur runs head-on to a wall, takes a step toward
the edge of the wall, followed by a Moon Step and a Crane Landing
on the top of the wall. This technique can be used to climb
up shoulder to head-high walls without using the hands.

Self-explanatory

English	French
Roll (4)/Rolling (3)/ Rolls (5)	Roulade (1, 3, 5)
Diving roll (4)	

Climbing (5)	Grimper (1)
Arm Jumps (5)/ Cat Leap (3,4)	Saut de bras (1,2,3,5)
Wall-up (3)/Wallrun (4)/ Wall Runs (5)	Passe muraille (1,2,3,5)
Small Wall-up (3)/ Wallhop (4)	Petit passe muraille (3)
Wall-up 360° (3)/ Wallhop 360° (4)	Passe muraille 360° (3)
	Planche (1,2)
Wall-up 360°	
Running Cat Leap (4)	
Level to Level Cat (4)	
Cat-to-Cat (5)	Retour de bras (5)

Explanation

The Parkour Roll is similar to the judo roll in that it is a rotation around
the diagonal axis. They are used to dissipate energy
(divert vertical energy into a rotational movement) when landing

Diving roll from an approach with distinct flight phase
(often used as a diving through technique)

Basic skill as a combination of moving up, climbing and supporting with a crossed-
synchronous pushing and pulling phase upward, downward and sideways

Jump onto an obstacle in the hanging position, landing on the feet on a vertical wall and
gripping the top edge or other place where obstacle can be gripped

Approach, one-footed take-off in front of the wall.
Step/stride onto a wall in order to gain height.
Support with the hands directly followed by tuck or crouch jump over chest
to head-height wall. Wall clearance with initial support by the feet
in the hanging position followed by lean *(planche)*.

See above, but smaller movement and clearance of a small wall

Step onto a vertical surface with 360° rotation around the longitudinal axis
(screw turn) directly followed by clearance *(planche)* of the wall

The lift can be performed from a hanging position (pull-up)
or after the arm jump with an overhand grip to support

Step/stride onto a wall with 360° rotation around the longitudinal axis,
then grip the wall edge

Running Arm Jump.

Arm Jump usually on a low or high level.

Arm Jump from a hanging position (Cat-Leap Position)
Or previous Arm Jump (combined with a push-off similar to Tic-Tac from
hanging position on vertical surface) with jump and a 180° longitudinal axis rotation to land
in a Cat Leap Position

English	French
Climbing (5)	Grimper (1)
Level to Level Cat	
Cat 180° (4)	
Cat 270° (4)	
Cat 360° (4)	
Swings and Hanging Movements (5)	Lâché (1, 2, 5)
Dyno (5)	Montée de bras (5)
Straight Lâché (5)	
Swinging Lâché (5)	
	Le balancer (2)
Underbar (4,5)/Clearing (5)	Franchissement (1, 2, 5, 6)
Feet First Underbar (5)	
Feet First Underbar to Precision	

Explanation

Basic skill as a combination of moving up, climbing and supporting with a crossed-synchronous pushing and pulling phase upward, downward and sideways

In a Level to Level Cat, the take-off is on the same level
as in the Cat Leap/Arm Jump landing. This means that one must jump down
into the Arm Jump position. Such a downward flight curve means
that the body has more momentum to absorb with the hands on landing,
but also that the feet/legs must absorb the energy,
which means that the feet cannot be optimally planted against the obstacle.

Once you are aware of this, as a solution you can
also let your feet slide down the wall, ending up hanging
with your hands on the edge of the wall. The obvious consequence
of this is that it is all the harder to pull yourself up afterwards,
but it does prevent a fall.

Arm Jump with a half rotation.

Quarter rotation from standing or hanging to hanging.

Complete turn before the actual landing in the Arm Jump.

Dropping from a hanging position

When climbing, fast powerful clearance technique using arms and legs

Simple drop from hanging position

Dropping from a swing (before or after legs are vertical)

Long hanging swing as swing technique for subsequent moves

Clearing obstacles in hanging position with or without (foot) contact on the lower part of the obstacle

A way of diving over a barrier in which the feet cross the barrier
before the hands make contact with it

English	French
Underbar (4,5)/Clearing (5)	Franchissement (1, 2, 5, 6)
Spiral Underbar (5)	
	Franchissement var
Spiral Underbar to Precision	

Freerunning Stunts/ Freerunning Elements/ Aerials & Flips	
Aerial (4)	
Axe to Aerial/ Reverse Aerial	
Aerial Twist	
Side Flip	
Side Flip Layout	
Wall Back Flip (4)	
Wall Back Flip/360°	
Wall Flip 360°	
Wall Flip 720°	
One Step Wall Flip/ Flash Kick	
Front Flip (4)	

Explanation

Clearing obstacles in a hanging position with or without (foot) contact
on the lower part of the obstacle

Clearance with additional help from the crossed grip
during take-off, ending with a twist over the obstacle

Acrobatic movements with rotations
around the horizontal and longitudinal axes

A free/unsupported somersault with legs in straddle position

Aerial preceded by backwards free leg kick from standing position

Aerial with rotation around the longitudinal axis

Flip to the side with take-off from lunge position and deployment of free leg
(see Aerial, page 214)

Extended Side Flip with legs in straddle position.
Side flip with opened and straight legs

Back flip with different leg positions (tucked, piked, straight)

Back flip from a push-off from a vertical or sloping wall

Back flip with a complete rotation

Wall Back flip with 720° rotation around the longitudinal axis

One step onto the wall is used to gain height
and to perform a fast, backwards wall flip

Forward flip with different leg positions (tucked, piked, straight)

English	French
Freerunning Stunts/ Freerunning Elements/ Aerials & Flips	
Handstand (4)	
Wall Spin (4)	
One Step Wall Spin	
Two Step Wall Spin	
Corner Wall Spin	

Sources:

1 = Kalteis, A. & Meyer, D. (2010) Parkour Grundbewegungen – Internet source.

2 = Parkour Association Germany (2010) Parkour – Techniques – Internet source.

3 = Sébastien, F. (2010) Freerunning Techniques – Internet source.

4 = Urban Free Flow (2010) Parkour/Freerun Techniques – Internet source.

5 = Edwards, D.(2009) *The Parkour & Freerunning Handbook*. London: Virgin Books.

6 = Luksch, M. (2009). *Tracers Blackbook. Geheimnisse der Parkour Technik*. Fisher Print.

Explanation

**Acrobatic movements with rotations
around the horizontal and longitudinal axes**

Handstand with extended body in the vertical position

Wall Spin with support on wall or similar vertical surface

One step onto the wall is used to gain height
and to lead into the vertical Wall Spin

Two steps onto the wall are used to gain height
and to lead into the vertical Wall Spin

Wall Spin over a wall corner

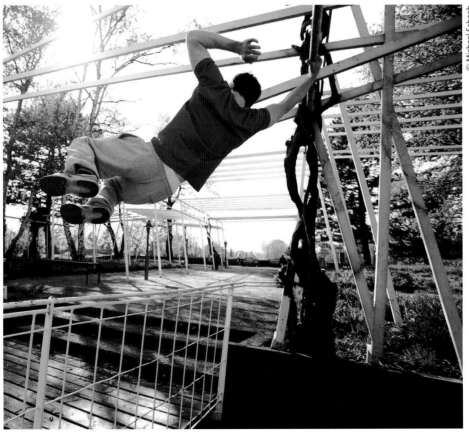

© Michael Schaab

9 BIBLIOGRAPHY

Archard, E. (1998, 1. Oktober). "Des hommes chat sur Bercy..." www.wmaker.net/parkour/Le-PARKOUR-by-DB_r8.html: l'équipe 1998 Bercy.jpg

Atkinson, M. (2009, 20. März). Parkour, anarcho-environmentalism, and poiesis. Loughborough University, UK. *Journal of Sport & Social Issues, Vol. 33,* Issue 2, p. 169, 26 p.

Bavinton, N. (2007). From obstacle to opportunity: Parkour, leisure, and the reinterpretation of constraints. Centre for Cultural Research, University of Western Sydney. *Annals of Leisure Research, Vol. 10,* Issue 3/4, 391.

Belle, J.-F. Internet Homepage of David Belle. www.kyzr.free.fr/davidbelle/

Belle, J.-F. (2006). Internet-Blog: "Official Blog Parkour by David Belle". Raymond Belle. www.wmaker.net/parkour/Raymond-Belle_r4.html

Blum, I. & Friedmann, K. (1994). *Trainingslehre – Sporttheorie für die Schule.* 4. Auflage. Pfullingen. Promos Verlag.

Blum, I. & Friedmann, K. (2001). *Trainingslehre – Sporttheorie für die Schule.* (Taschenbuch). Pfullingen. Promos Verlag.

Cometti, G. (1988). *La Pliométrie.* Dijon. Univ. de Bourgogne.

Crowell, H. P., Treadwell, T. A., Faughn, J. A., Leiter, K. L., Woodward, A. A., Yates, C.E. (1995). Lower Extremity Assistance for parachutists (LEAP) Program: Quantification of the biomechanics of the the parachute landing fall and implications for a device to prevent injuries. Aberdeen Proving Ground: *U.S. Army research Laboratory,* Report No.: ARL-TR-926.

De Marées, H. (2003). *Sportphysiologie.* Köln. Sportverlag Strauß.

Desbois, G. (1999, Oktober). „David Belle et le Parcours, une histoire de la famille". "Official Blog Parkour by David Belle" www.wmaker.net/parkour/Le-PARKOUR-by-DB_r8.html?start=3: david belle le parcours2.jpg

Devita, P. & Skelly, W. (1992). Effect of landing stiffness on joint kinetics and energetics in the lower extremity. *Medicine and Science in Sports and Exercise, Vol. 24,* No. 1, 108-115.

Dufek, J. S. & Bates, B.T. (1990). The evaluation and prediction of impact forces during landings. *Medicine and Science in Sports and Exercise Vol. 22,* No.1, 370-377.

Edwards, D. (2009). *Parkour.* New York: Crabtree Publishing Company.

Edwards, D. (2009). *The parkour and freerunning handbook.* London: Virgin Books.

Ehlenz, H., Grosser, M. & Zimmermann, E. (1985[2]). *Krafttraining.* München – Wien – Zürich: BLV Verlagsgesellschaft.

Fend, H. (2000). Qualität und Qualitätssicherung im Bildungswesen. *Zeitschrift für Pädagogik, 41.* Beiheft. 55-72.

Foucan, S. (2008). Internet homepage – *Foucan Story – background & history*.
    www.foucan.com/?page_id=19

Foucan, S. (2008). Internet homepage – *freerunning academie – freerunning techniques*. unter
    www.foucan.com/?page_id=34

Freiwald, J. (2009). *Optimales Dehnen – Sport, Prävention, Rehabilitation*. Balingen, Spitta
    Verlag.

Friedmann, K. (2008). *Trainingslehre – Sporttheorie für die Schule*. Pfullingen: Promos Verlag.

Fukunage, T. (1976). Die absolute Muskelkraft und das Muskeltraining. *Sportarzt und
    Sportmedizin, 27*, 255-265.

Gaulhofer, K. & Streicher, M. (1930/31). *Natürliches Turnen. Gesammelte Aufsätze*.
    Bd. I, II. Wien/Leipzig.

Gerling, I. E. (2009). *Teaching Children's Gymnastics*. 2nd Edition. Maidenhead. Meyer &
    Meyer Sports (UK) Ltd.

Gerling, I. E. (2011). *Basisbuch Gerätturnen*. 7. überarb. Auflage. Aachen. Meyer & Meyer
    Sportverlag.

Gerling, I. E. (2012). *Gerätturnen für Fortgeschrittene – Band 1: Boden und Schwebebalken*. 3.
    Auflage. Aachen. Meyer & Meyer Sportverlag.

Gerling, I. E. (2008). *Gerätturnen für Fortgeschrittene – Band 2: Sprung-, Hang- und
    Stützgeräte*. Aachen. Meyer & Meyer Sportverlag.

Gissel, N. & Schwier, J. (Hrsg.). (2003). *Abenteuer, Erlebnis und Wagnis. Perspektiven für
    den Sport in der Schule und Verein?* Tagungsband 134 zur Jahrestagung der
    dvs-Sektion Sportpädagogik vom 30.5.-1.6.2002 in Gießen. Hamburg: Czwalina
    Verlag.

Göring, A. & Lutz, M. (2008). Le Parkour – Zwischen Trend und Tradition. *Landes-sportbund
    Niedersachsen. Nr. 4*, 16-17; Nr. 5, 22-23.

Grosser, M., Brüggemann, P. & Zintl, F. (1986). *Leistungssteuerung in Training und Wettkampf*.
    München-Wien-Zürich. BLV Verlagsgesellschaft.

Grosser, M. (1991). *Schnelligkeitstraining. Grundlagen, Methoden, Leistungssteuerung,
    Programme*. BLV Verlagsgesellschaft, München.

Heinlin, C. (2008). Parkour – l'art de déplacement. *Sport Praxis, Jg. 49*, Heft 11, Wiebelsheim,
    Limpert Verlag.

Hébert, G. (1912). *Méthode naturelle*. Paris

Hébert, G. (1912/1934). *L'éducation physique on l'entraînement complet par la méthode
    naturelle – Exposé et resultats*. Paris: Librairie Vuibert.

Hess, M. & Hess, S. (2007). *Parkour Association Germany*. Internet Homepage. Zugriff am 17.
    Februar 2010 unter www.myparkour.de/

Hirtz, P., Hotz, A. & Ludwig, G. (2000). *Gleichgewicht*. Schorndorf. Verlag Karl Hofmann.

Ide, J. (2007). Von der Hasenheide zum Freerunning. *NTB-Magazin, 06*, 18.

Jahn, F. L. & Eiselen, E. (1816): *Die Deutsche Turnkunst zur Einrichtung der Turnplätze.* Berlin.

Kalteis, A. (2006, 3. März). *Le Parkour Austria. Artikel: Fallen/Landen.* Zugriff am 11.7.2009 unter www.le-parkour.at/fond.html

Kalteis, A. & Meyer, D. (keine Angaben zum Zeitpunkt der Veröffentlichung). *Le Parkour Austria. Artikel: Parkour Grundbewegungen.* Zugriff am 9.7.2009 unter www.le-parkour.at/grund.html

Knebel, K.-P. (2005). *Muskelcoaching: Top in Form mit Streching. Richtig dehnen. Mehr leisten. Verletzungen vorbeugen.* Reinbeck. Rowohlt Taschenbuch Verlag.

Krick, F. (2008). Le Parkour oder die Kunst der Fortbewegung. *Sportpädagogik, Heft 4/5,* 44-53.

Krüger, M. (2002). Der Streit um das "richtige" Turnen. In M. Roscher (Hrsg.), *Gerätturnen: eine Bewegungskultur in der Diskussion.* (S. 9-31). Hamburg. Czwalina Verlag.

Kurz, D. (1992). Sport mehrperspektivisch unterrichten – warum und wie? In K. Zieschang & W. Buchmeier (Hrsg.), *Sport zwischen Tradition und Zukunft.. (Bericht über den ...Kongress des Ausschusses Deutscher Leibeserzieher (ADL; 11) (S. 15-18),* Schorndorf: Hofmann Verlag. Postprint frei zugänglich unter www.repositories.ub.uni-bielefeld.de/biprints/volltexte/2009/1755URN: urn:nbn:de:0070-bipr-17555

Kurz, D. (2009). *Vom Sinn des Sports.* Abschiedvorlesung, 27.1.2009. Universität Bielefeld. Internet Homepage, Zugriff am 7.4.2010. Download unter www.schulsport-nrw.de/info/news08/pdf/d_kurz_vom_sinn_des_sports.pdf

Lassleben, A. (2007). Tic-Tac und Wallspin – Anregungen für den Trendsport Parkour. *Sportpädagogik, Heft 4/5, Heft 5,* 41-43.

Liedtke, S. (2009). "Le parkour" & Freerunning – Hindernisse kreativ überwinden im Schulsport. *Betrifft Sport. Nr. 3,* 10-13.

Liedtke, S. (2009). Von "basic moves" zum ersten „run"! *Betrifft Sport, Nr. 4,* 19-31.

Lindemann, U. (2009). Le Parkour im Schulsport – Und was ist mit der Sicherheit? *Betrifft Sport, Nr. 4,* 7-11.

Luksch, M. (2009). *Tracers Blackbook – Geheimnisse der Parkourtechnik.* Fisher Print.

Marinsek, M. (2010). Basic landing characteristics and their application in artistic gymnastics. *Science Gymnastics Journal Vol 2,* No. 2, 59-67.

McNitt-Gray, J. L. (1991). Kinetics and impulse characteristics of during drop landings from three heights. *Int. J. Sport Biomech. 7,* 201-204.

McNitt-Gray, J. L. (1993). Kinetics of the lower extremities during drop landings from three heights. *Journal of Biomechanics Vol. 26,* No. 9, 1037-1046.

Meyer, D. (2007, 3. November). *Parkour.NET – the official Parkour Portal powered by Traceurs, for Traceurs.*

Mizrahi, J. & Suzak, Z. (1982). Analysis of parameters affecting impact force attenuation during landing in human vertical free fall. *Engineering in Medicine Vol. 11,* No. 3, 141-147

Müller, A. (2009, 20. März). *Freerunning.net. Bewegungskünste. Parkour. David Belle.* Zugriff am 16.3.2010 unter www.freerunning.net/de/community/lexikon/david-belle

Pape-Kramer, S. & Heinlin, C. (2007). Le Parkour. *Sportunterricht. Jg. 56*, Heft 6, 169-175; 191-192.

Peters, W. (2009). *Abitur: Training – Sport – Trainingslehre – Grundlagen und Auf-gaben mit Lösungen – Leistungskurs* (aktualisierte/neu überarbeitete Auflage). Freising. Stark Verlagsgesellschaft.

Pette, D. (1999). Das adaptive Potential des Skelettmuskels. *Deutsche Zeitschrift für Sportmedizin, 50*, 262-271.

Rochhausen, S. (2009). *Parkoursport im Schulturnen.* (2. Auflage). Norderstedt, Books on Demand. www.parkoursport.de

Schiffer, J. (1993). *Schnelligkeit – trainingsmethodische, biomechanische, leistungs-physiologische und leistungsdiagnostische Aspekte. Eine kommentierte Bibliographie.* Sport und Buch Strauß. *Edition Sport.* Köln.

Schmidtbleicher, D. & Gollhofer, A. (1985). Einflußgrößen des reaktiven Bewegungsver-haltens und deren Bedeutung für die Sportpraxis. In: Buhrle, M. (Hrsg.): Grundlagen des Maximal- und Schnellkrafttrainings. *Schriftenreihe des Bundesinstituts für Sportwissenschaft, Bd. 56.* Schorndorf. Verlag Karl Hofmann. 271-281.

Schulz, A. (2009). Unterrichtsvorhaben – Le Parkour, erste Erfahrungen mit dem Überwinden von Hindernissen in einer fünften Klasse. *Betrifft Sport, Nr. 4,* 12-18.

Tuccaro, A. (1599/1987). *Trois Dialogues.* A Reproduction of the Copy in the British Library. Archival Facsimiles Limited. Alburgh (Erstausgabe in Paris 1599).

Urban Free Flow Ltd. (2008, 24. Dezember). Veröffentlichung: *Sébastien Foucan: Interview.* www.urbanfreeflow.com/2008/12/24/sebastien-foucan-interview

Weineck, J. (2007). *Optimales Training – Leistungsphysiologische Trainingslehre unter besonderer Berücksichtigung des Kinder- und Jugendtrainings.* (15. Auflage) Balingen. Spitta Verlag.

Whitting, J. W., Steele, J. R., Jafrey, M. A., Munro, B. J. (2007). Parachute landing fall characteristics at three realistic vertical descent velocities. *Aviation, Space and Environmental Medicine Vol. 78*, No. 12, 1135-1142.

Witfeld, J. (2010). *Zum Einfluss von Höhe, Weite und Landetechnik auf die mechanischen Belastungen im Knie- und Sprunggelenk in der Sportart Parkour.* Diplomarbeit. Köln: Deutsche Sporthochschule Köln, Deutschland.

Wolters, P., Ehni, H., Kretschmer, J., Scherler, K. & Weichert, W. (2000). *Didaktik des Schulsports.* Schorndorf. Verlag Karl Hofmann.

ACKNOWLEDGEMENTS

I would like to thank all my friends who have contributed to this book project.

Firstly, I'd like to thank Ilona Gerling who first made this book possible and whose experience has enriched and guided its contents. My thanks also go to Marc P Dresson and Alexander Pach and the whole coaching team of Move Artistic. Together, we have tried to summarize what we have been working on in recent years in countless workshops and training sessions. Guys, this book contains our experiences and contributions. I would like to personally highlight the time I spent with Kirill Seleznev and Paul Jung. So many ideas, layouts and methodological reflections have originated from our collaborative college coaching work.

I also owe special thanks to Michael Schaab. Your outdoor photos have made this book into a real work of art. Thank you for the many photo shoots you set up with Paul J., Kirill S., Frauke Meyn and me, and for your commitment to this book project.

At the risk of not naming all my friends, I would like to finish by thanking Jonathan Haehn for his quick preparation of the layout diagrams.

I would like to dedicate this book to my parents and my wife Lu. Thank you for your support. You have enabled me to follow my goals and have supported and accompanied me all the way, making this book possible in the first place. Thank you for always being there for me.

Jan Witfeld

APPENDIX 1

In September 2009, American Parkour began a community effort to define Parkour. They invited the entire community to post their personal definition of Parkour. It was edited into the final version by a committee of American Parkour employees and people outside of American Parkour to ensure that it was truly a community effort.

Their result:

- Parkour is the physical discipline of training to overcome any obstacle within one's path by adapting one's movements to the environment.
- Parkour requires: consistent, disciplined training with an emphasis on functional strength, physical conditioning, balance, creativity, fluidity, control, coordination, precision, spatial awareness, and looking beyond the traditional use of objects.
- Parkour movements typically include: running, jumping, vaulting, climbing, balancing, and quadrupedal movement. Movements from other physical disciplines are often incorporated, but acrobatics or tricking alone do not constitute parkour.
- Parkour training focuses on: safety, longevity, personal responsibility, and self-improvement. It discourages reckless behavior, showing off, and dangerous stunts.
- Parkour practitioners value: community, humility, positive collaboration, sharing of knowledge, and the importance of play in human life, while demonstrating respect for all people, places, and spaces.

American Parkour Community Definition[1]

One of the American Parkour Federations is the **World Freerunning Parkour Federation (WFPF)**. The WFPF recognized the need in the U.S. for a structured conditioning and training program to make Parkour broadly accessible to people of all fitness levels, ages, genders, and sizes. MOVE is a fitness program designed to improve an individual's ability to navigate through the world with power, efficiency, and confidence. Based on the movements of Parkour, MOVE is designed to develop, through structured conditioning and training, the human body's natural movements from point "A" to point "B", making it a truly functional approach that is broadly applicable and benefical to anyone interested in improving their level of fitness. Through the development of the body's natural movements, MOVE also facilitates and nurtures an improved mind-body connection, bringing the practitioner more in touch with his or her physical and mental capabilities, increasing confidence and encouraging individuals to see their world in a new way.

[1] American Parkour. "American Parkour: What is Parkour?".

americanparkour.com. http://www.americanparkour.com/whatisparkour.

APPENDIX 2

LANDING STRESSES – SCIENTIFIC FINDINGS

In the following chapter we want to provide a brief overview of biomechanical research studies on the subject of 'landing'. In conclusion, we will introduce a further biomechanical comparative study of the different landing techniques in Parkour.

INTRODUCTION

A landing can be seen as a collision between the body and the ground in which the body exerts forces on the ground, and external forces known as ground reaction forces are exerted on the body. These ground reaction forces lead to mechanical stress of the musculoskeletal system and therefore inevitably stress the biological structures (such as muscles, tendons, cartilage, meniscus, bone).

REMINDER:

When biological structures are put under stress, this can lead to tissue adaptations that improve mechanical physical properties (e.g., muscle building) or to physical damage or breakdown (e.g., injuries).

Ground reaction forces can be quantified by special measuring equipment and represented as force-time curves (compare force-time curves on p.315). The ground reaction forces are determined by different factors: on the one hand they are influenced by the kinetic energy of the body on impact and the chosen landing technique and on the other hand by the type of ground surface.

In order to keep the stress on the musculoskeletal system as low as possible, biomechanical research is trying to identify ways of reducing the maximal forces exerted and ensure optimal energy absorption by the musculature.

Which biomechanical findings can help to keep landing stress in Parkour as low as possible?

Parkour landings are usually onto hard surfaces, so that the best way of influencing ground reaction forces is by the choice of landing technique.

The choice of an appropriate landing technique should be anticipated already before take-off. Maximum ground reaction forces already occur a few milliseconds after initial ground contact (touchdown), especially when jumping from heights. They are also termed passive forces because they cannot be controlled by muscle reflexes. To respond specifically to these immediate impact forces, the chosen landing technique must already be anticipated prior to contact with the ground. This is reflected already during the flight by an early activation of the muscles involved in landing.

Increased speed on impact (e.g., from greater heights) leads to a requirement for a stronger pre-activation of the muscles.

On a landing, both the agonistic as well as the antagonistic working of the muscles is in the form of a co-contraction. The type of muscle activation determines the landing technique. In turn, the landing technique has a decisive influence on the ground reaction forces and the forces acting on the body (internal forces).

Research findings on jumping down have shown that two-foot landings can most effectively reduce maximal ground reaction forces and allow more energy to be absorbed by the musculature than one-foot landings. In addition, it can be shown that soft two-foot landings on the feet with high joint flexion in the ankles, knees and hips (compared to stiff landings) have the potential to reduce peak ground reaction forces even more and allow the muscles to absorb more of the body's kinetic energy.

This principle can be compared to the way an airbag works, which also reduces peak impact forces by prolonging the impact phase.

Mats and shock absorption soles also work according to the same function principle. It has been shown that mats can reduce the peak ground reaction forces and change the distribution of internal forces. However it has also been established that probands in laboratory research adapted their landing techniques to the landing surface. Mats, for example, lead to landings with low joint flexion and therefore to higher peak forces than would have been the case with soft landings on mats.

But what about the stresses with the special Parkour landing techniques carried out in connection with follow-on movements (e.g., landing & rolling or landing & diverting)?

In a comparison of level landings and landings with subsequent rolling motion, Mizrahi & Susak noted as early as 1982 that there were less maximum ground reaction forces during landings with rolling movements.

In a more recent bio-mechanical diploma thesis study in 2010 at the German Sport University Cologne (Witfeld, 2010) a comparison was made of standing landings and landings with divert movements, the landings usual in Parkour.

The following describes the study into Parkour landing techniques and then shows the results of the investigation.

Title: The influence of height, width, and landing techniques on the mechanical stresses to the knee and ankle joints in the sport of Parkour

INTRODUCTION

In the Parkour and Free Running scene, jump landings with follow-on rolling movements as opposed to silent landings (standing) are described as a more effective landing technique to reduce stress on the joints of the lower extremities. A comparative biomechanical stress analysis and analysis of three different landing techniques for jumping in the sport of Parkour was used to examine this thesis.

EXECUTION

Ten experienced Traceurs or freerunners took part in a laboratory study to examine the influence of landing techniques, jump height and width on the mechanical stresses. The probands carried out landings in a standing position (LS), landings with rolling motion (LR) and landings with diverts (LD) (cf. sequences pp.313f) from two different jump heights (1.17 m, 1.95 m) with three different width distances (0.5 m, 1.5 m, 2.65 m).

The ground reaction forces were determined by using a force plate (1,250 Hz). A three-dimensional motion caption system (Vicon Nexus, 250 Hz) was used for the analysis of the landing techniques This analysis system allowed the creation of an individual body model of each of the probands (see Figure: Body model). Each landing could therefore be analyzed by using this in combination with the force plate.

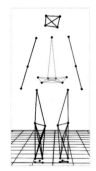

Figure: Body Model of a proband standing

The mechanical stresses were examined on the basis of the horizontal and vertical ground reaction forces, the external joint moments, the impulses of the external joint moments, as well as joint performance and joint work in the knee and the ankle.

The quantification of the joint moments and joint performance of knee and ankle joints was carried out by inverse dynamic calculations (MATLAB) in the sagittal plane. The kinematic motion analysis and the mechanical stress analysis were carried out within a time interval of 150 ms after initial contact with the ground, because within this time frame the largest strains were suspected.

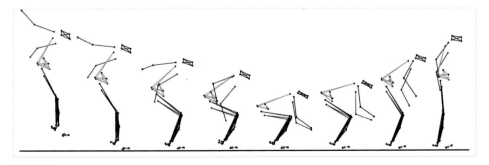

Sequence of a landing (standing) by a proband jumping from a height of 1.95m and for a width of 1.5m

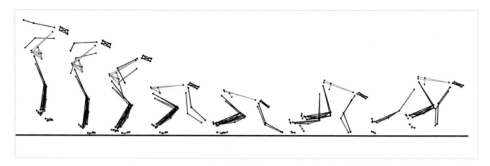

Sequence of a divert landing by a proband jumping from a height of 1.95m and for a width of 1.5m

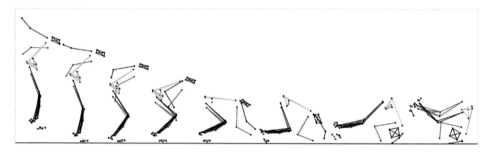

Sequence of landing with a rolling motion by a proband jumping from a height of 1.95m and for a width of 1.5m

RESEARCH RESULTS

The significant difference in the ground reaction forces consisted of a distinct difference in the horizontal brake impulse of the ground reaction forces. The standing landings showed the largest horizontal braking impulses, the landings with rolling motion (LR) the smallest braking impulses and the landings with deflection (LD) half way between both. This phenomenon can be explained by the various landing techniques. In a standing landing, the speed of the body's center of gravity must be brought to a standstill during the two-footed touchdown phase. In contrast, with the two other landing techniques, it is already anticipated that after a two-footed landing there is a subsequent follow-on movement. In addition to the mentioned differences of the horizontal brake impulses, the anticipation of an additional movement had, among other things, an effect on the peak horizontal and vertical force values of the ground reaction forces. In landings with a rolling motion (LR) and the landings with deflection (LD), the peak horizontal and vertical force values were significantly lower than in standing landings.

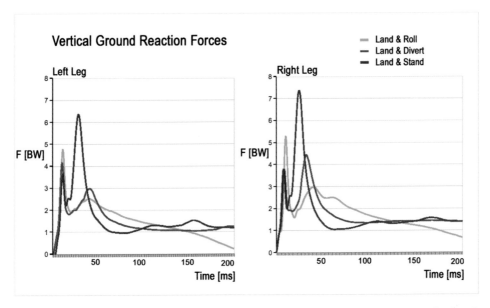

Example force-time curves of the vertical ground reaction forces for the three different landing techniques (land & roll, land & divert, land & stand) of a proband from a height of 1.95m with a width of 1.50m. The unit of force is [BW] (bodyweight) and the unit of time is [ms].

The research results of the ankle joint kinetics (the internal forces at the ankle) have shown that in landings with a rolling motion (following a two-footed landing) more power must be applied from the ankle than in standing landings. This, presumably, is a result of a landing on the balls of the feet in conjunction with a greater extent of movement at the ankle joint. However, it can be stated that the ability of the ankle to absorb energy was comparable for all landing techniques. The main difference could be observed in the knee joint.

In landings with rolling motion, significantly more force must be applied from the muscles involved in the movement of the knee joint and passive structures than in the two other landing techniques. Through the increased development of force of the knee joint muscles, increased tension on the tendons can be assumed, especially on the patellar tendon. However, significantly higher absorption of energy in landings with a rolling motion was measured in the knee muscles compared to the two other landing techniques. In comparison, in standing landings, less force had to be applied to the knee joint - it also absorbed the least energy.

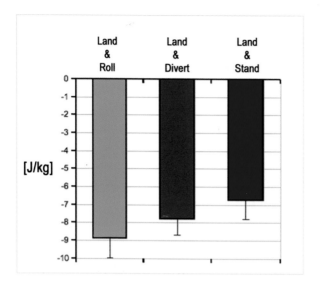

Bar chart (and standard deviations) of the negative work of the knee joints (sum of the left and right legs) of 10 probands (traceurs/freerunners) in a jump from a height of 1.95m with a jumping distance of 1.50m in intervals of 150ms after the initial impact.

Negative knee joint work can be seen as an indicator of how much energy is absorbed by the muscles involved in the knee action in a specific period of time.

This result raised the question how the kinetic energy in standing landings was absorbed, because the center of gravity of the body in standing landings – in contrast to landings with follow-on movements – must be brought to a standstill and this can only be achieved by absorption of the entire kinetic energy involved.

It is assumed that the body position for the touchdown has a particular influence on the internal forces in the knee. A larger lever between force vector of the ground reaction forces and center of the joint causes greater joint moments and promotes the energy absorption of the joint muscles. A force vector that cuts close or passes through the knee joint at the knee joint center complicates a muscular response and increases the compression forces within the knee joint. In addition, a smaller lever leads to a lower absorption of energy and by contrast, this results in a greater absorption of energy by deformation in the knee (of bone, cartilage, and meniscus).

According to this conclusion, it can be assumed that, because of the position of the body on touchdown and the requirement to create a greater braking force, the lower limbs must be braced even against the ground. This means that less energy can be absorbed by the muscles in the knee joint and more energy is absorbed due to compression or deformation of the biological structures than landings with follow-on movements.

SUMMARY AND CONCLUSION

The results of this study suggest that the landings with subsequent roll motion (LR), as well as divert landings (LD) – as used in the sport of Parkour – hold the potential to reduce the peak force values of the ground reaction forces and absorb more energy through the knee muscles than in soft standing landings. In a land and roll type of landing a stronger creation of force in the ankle and knee joint muscles was detectable that is likely to cause greater tension on the Achilles and patellar tendon.

The probands in this study had many years' training experience and can be described as landing experts. For less experienced people or athletes, these landing techniques with follow-on movements are certainly a more difficult challenge on their coordinative and muscular abilities.

However, for the learning process it seems advisable to focus first on practicing different kinds of landing on different surfaces. The training goal should initially focus on carrying out soft, two-foot, ball-heel standing landings combined with a wide range of movement in the joints and focus on a deliberate, correct joint action (so-called stiff landings with knock knees should be avoided).

A foundation of a diverse landing training of typical Parkour landing techniques with follow-on movements appears to be a proven means of reducing the peak force values in drop landings and allowing the muscles of the knee to absorb more energy.

INDEX

180° Cat 83

270° Cat 83

360° Cat 83

360° passe muraille 83

A

Abilities, Coordination 52, 54, 61 90

Abilities, Strength 56-57, 61, 63-64

Ability, Balance 52, **85-88**, 90-91

Ability, Coordination 54, 61

Ability, Coupling 53

Ability, Differentiation 52

Ability, Orientation 52, 90

Ability, Rhythmization 52

Absoption of energy 315-316

Adaptation Processes, physical 48

Advanced Moves 84, **213-239**

Adventure 255-256, 258, 260

Aerial 84, **214-222**, 282, 300, 302

Aerobic Capacity 41

Anaerobic capacity 41

Anatomy 39

Arm Jumps .... 35, 73, 83, 85, 99, 101, ... 177, **186-191**, 259, 274, 293, 295-299

Arroyo, Daniel 11

ATP **45-47**, 58, 60, 65

ATP/CP 45-47

Axes of Rotation 282

Axis, bent 282

Axis, sagittal .... 214, 216, ... 222, 226, 229, 232, 282

Axis, transversal 282

B

Back flip .... 84, 213, 234, 236, ... 259, 276-277, 291, 300-301

Balance 51-52, 75-76, 82, **85-91**, 109, 121, 259, 288, 298, 309

Balancing .... 20, 22, 27, 29, 35-36, ... 50, 72, 81, 84, **85-92**, ... 259-262, 264, 273-274, 289, 309

Balancing on All Fours (Cat Balance) 89-90

Balancing on the feet 88

Balancing on the hands
(Handstand) 41, 75, 82,
.... 87, **90-94**, 130, 259,
.... 281, 288-289, 302-303

Balancing, dynamic 87

Behavior, General 33-34

Belle, David 10, **19-28**, 31-33, 250

Benefits 73, 87, 258, 268

Bent Axis 282

C

Calf muscles 63, 76

Carbohydrates 43-46

Cartwheel 217-218, 220, 226

Cat Balance 89-90

Cat Leap 36, 73, 78, 83, 85, 98-101,
.... 147, 164, 168, 177, **186-191**,
.... 195-196, 259, 274, 291, 293, 296-299

Cat Path 292

Cat Walking 288

Cat-to-Cat 98, 296

Clearing 26, 81, 84, 94, 145,
.... 189, 201, 208, 263, 269,
.... 272, 275, 278, 291, 298-301

Climbing 27, 35, 51, 73,

.... 78-79, 81, 84-85, 89,
..... **177-179**, 194, 259-262, 296-299, 309

Climb-up 192

Clothing **36-37**, 252

Competitions 28, 244-247, 252

Composition of Parkour 259

Concentric 41, 56

Cool Down 70, **73**, 269

Cooperation 32, 51, 258, 272, 276-277

Coordination 27, 40, 41, 51-73,
.... 91, 266, 309

Coordination, Intramuscular .. 40, 57-62, 66

Core Training 74-79

Corner Wall Spin 227, 302

Courir 94-96

Crane 82, 113, **115-117**, 290-295

Crane Moon Step 117, 294

Creatine Phosphate (CP) . 45-47, 58, 60, 65

Culbuter 213

Curriculum Structure 260

D

Dash Bomb 153, 292

Dash Vault 83, **152-156**, 158, 201,
.... 275-276, 292-293

Definition of Freerunning 26

Definition of Parkour 25, **26**

Demi-tour 83, 166-172, 290, 292

Des Sauts de Précision 105-111

Dismount 82, 148-149, 164, 169,
.... 172, 177, 183-184, 194-196,
.... 220, 288, 294

Diverting, landing **122-124**, 128, 312

Diving Kong 83, **144**, 292

Diving Roll 82, **130**, 296-297

Doyle, Ryan 242-249

Drinking 44

Drop 82, 87, 97, **112**, 118,
.... 122-130, 133, 141, 166, 183,
.... 194, 197, 261, 264, 288,
.... 290, 294, 299, 317

Dynamic Balancing 87

Dynamic Stretching 67, **68**, 72

Dyno 83, 298

E

Eccentric 41, 56, 113, 118-121,
.... 123, 147

Eccentric Silent Landing 113, 118, 123

Endurance 31, 41, 50-51, 54-57,
.... 63-65, 73, 75, 96, 269, 272

Endurance, Strength 51, 55-57, 63-64

Energy supply 39, **42-46**, 57, 63, 70

Enviroment 23, 25-26, 31-32, 34,
...51-52, 73, 241, 253, 255, 260, 266, 309

Equilibré 85, 288

Excitement 255-256, 258

Expression 255, 257, 258

F

Fairness 258

Fast-twitch fibers **41-42**, 57, 65-66

Fatigue 41, 46, 49, 55, 66, 96

Fats 43-44

Fitness 50, 66, 71, 112, 255,
.... 257-258, 309

Flag 84, 259, 288

Flash Kick 235, 300

Flexibility 51-52, **67-74**

Flight balance 87

Foucan, Sébastian 10, 14, 19, 23,
.... **24-26**, 27-28, **31-32**,

Franchissement 201, 299-300

Freerunner ... 10, 14, 27, 28, 33, 35-37, 74,
.... 241, 250-253, 255, 266, 282, 312

Freerunning values 31-32

Fun 11, 66, 73, 249, 250

G

General Behavior 33-34

Gerling, Ilona E. 15-17, 308

Glossary of techniques 288-303

Glycogen reserve 45-47

Grimper 177, 296-299

Grip, Mixed 284, 287, 291

Grip, Overhand 78, 92, 283, 286, 297

Grip, Underhand 78, 284, 286-287

Gripe, Spokebone 283

Grips 283-287

Gustaffson, Markus 242-249

H

Handstand 41, 75, 82, 87, **90-94**, 130,
.... 259, 281, 288-289, 302-303

Hang Grips 283-287

Hanging 73, 77-78, 81, 83,
.... **197-200**, 259, 294-301

Health 31, 33-34, 252-253,
.... 255, 257-258, 269

Heart Rate 55

Hébert, Georges 19-22, 25

Historical development 19-29

Hynh, Khoa 242-249

I

Indoor Training 28, 34-35, 244

Interval 313, 316

Intramuscular Coordination ... 40, 57-62, 66

J

Jumping forms 97

Jumps 41, 63, 76-77, 82-83,
....................................**97-112**, 259, 288-297

Jump, Running 97, 100, 210,
.... 274, 288-289

Jumps, supported 291-295

K

Kash Vault 83, **156-157**, 283, 292

Kilby, Sam 11

Kocsis, A`bel 213

Kong to Cat 83, 147, 292

Kong to Precision .... 83, 145, 151 , 292

Kong Vault 81, 83, 98, 125, 130,
.... **144-151**, 156, 259, 282, 292-293

L

Lâché 83, **197-200**, 298

Landing 41, 76, 81-84, 81, 97, 99,
.... **113-130**, 259, 261, 264, 267,
.... 288-299, 310-317

Landing and Diverting 122, 124

Landing and jog away 259, 291, 293

Landing Basics 82, 113, 294

Landing in Lunge Position 113-114

Landing Strategy . 113, 124, 126, 162-163

Landing Stresses 310-317

Landing Techniques 113-114, 126, 264,
.... 310-317

Lateral Vault 290

Lazy Gainer 141, 290

Lazy to Drop 141, 290

Lazy Vault 72, 140, 290

Le balancer 298

Leroux, Yoann 12

Lesson plans, PK in schools 269-278

Level to Level Cat 188, 296, 298-299

Loading Duration 54-55

Loops 84

M

Méthode Naturelle 19-20, 25

Methodical Principles 53

Monkey 83, **144**, 197, 259, 286, 292

Montée de bras 83, 298

Mounts 83

Movement Balancing 90

Muscle Cells 44-45, 65

Muscle Fiber Types 41

Muscle-up 78, 177, **192-193**

N

Nerve-muscle sytem 57-58, 64

Nunez, Gabriel 242-249

Nutrition **42-48**, 50

Nutritional Rules 42-43

O

One step wall flip 235, 300

One-foot Precision 106-107

Outdoor rules 266

Outdoor Training 35

P

Pach, Alex 241

Palm Spin 83, **172-176**, 294-295

Parkour Roll 118, 282, 297

Passe barrriére 82, **130**, 290-294

Passe Muraille 83, **179**, 296

Passement (Lazy) 82, **140-143**

Passement arriére 83, **162-166**, 292

Passement Assis 83, **152-156**, 292

Passement de chat 83, 292

Passement Rapide **134**, 290

Passement speed 83, 292

Paul, Jason 10, 242-249

Peak Forces 312

Pedagogical Aims 255

Petit passe murraille 83, 296

Philosophy of PK & FR 14-15, 19-25,
.... 31, 33, 250

Physical Experience 255, 257-258, 269

Physiology 39

Planche 83, 192, 296-297

Posture 39, 41, 92, 191, 239

Precision jumps 35, 72, 82, 97,
.... **105-111**, 120-121, 131, 288-289

Precision, One-foot 106-107

Precision, running 110-111, 288

Precision, Two-foot 108-109

Proteins 43

Q

Quadriceps, muscles 63, 92

Quadrupédie 82, 288

R

Rationales for PK in Schools 255

Reactive Jumping Exercise 63, 77

Réception **113-130**, 294

Red skeletal muscle fibers 41

Regaining a state of static balance 87-88

Retour de bras 296

Réverse 83, 162, 292

Reverse to cat 292

Reverse Vault **162-166**, 292

Risk 33-36, 54-55, 60, 67,
... 70-71, 89, 241, 255-256, 258, 260-261

Roll 36, 72, 81, 82, 87, 113, 118,
.... **126-130**, 259, 282, 289,
.... 296-297, 311-317

Roulade 126, 296

Running 84, 94-96, 259

S

Safety 29, **31-37**, 213, 260,
.... 264-265, 309

Safety Measures 34, 213

Saut á làrrêt 288

Saut d`élan 288

Saut de Bras 85, **186-188**, 296

Saut de Chat 98, 130, **144**, 292

Saut de détente 288

Saut de précision 288

Sauts de Fond **112**, 118

Scarlett, Ethan 12

School 20-21, 29, 35, 39,
.... 231, 251, 253, **255-278**

Sensation 257, 258

Sequence of Parkour 259

Shieff, Tim 10, 13

Shoes **35-37**, 51, 239, 252

Side Flip **221-225**, 282, 300-301

Skeletal Musculature 39

Slow-twitch-fibers **41-42**, 57

Speed 29, 31, 51, **64-66**, 75, 259, 311

Speed Vault **134-139**, 292

Spiral underbar to precisions 209, 300

Spotting 35, 92, 258, 264-265

Landing, Staggered 294

Standing Jump 87, 288

Static Balancing 85-87

Static Stretching 67-68, 70-74

Step Vault 72, **132-134**, 290

Stepping Movements 98, 290

Straight Landing 294-295

Strength 19, 29, 31, 41, 42,
.... 48-55, **56-64**, 74-78, 85, 90,
.... 184, 192, 269, 270, 309

Strength Endurance 51, 55-57, 63-64

Strength, Maximal 51, 56-58, **61-64**, 71-72

Strength performance 56-61, 72

Strength, Reactive 56-59, 62-65

Strength, Speed 42, 47, 51, 54,
.... 56-58, 61-64, 68

Stretching 48, 60, **67-69**, 70-74, 267

Stretching Training 41

Supplementary Training 74-79

Support 29, 34-35, 41, 51, 53, 81,
.... 85-87, 132, 255, 259, 268,
.... 283, 285, 291-303

Support grips (Spotting grips) 147, 285

Support Jumps 97, 98, 114,
.... 123, 162, 291-295

Swinging 51, 78, 81, 84,
.... **197-199**, 259, 298

T

Take-off 41, 76, 94, **97-103**,
.... 106, 109-110, 259, 289-301

Technique Training 52-53, 244

Tension 40-41, 60, 67, 70-71,
.... 77-78, 86, 92, 315, 317

Tic-Tac 82, **97-104**, 259, 276,
.... 290-291, 297

Traceur 14, 26, 33, 35-37,
.... 51, 74, 241, 250, 252-253,
.... 255, 266, 281

Training Frequency 55

Training Rules **34**, 48

Training, Intramuscular coordination 40,
.... 57-62, 66

Training, Muscle building 58-61, 64, 310

Transversal Axis 282

Turn Vault 72, 83, **166-171**, 292

Turning balance 87

Two-foot Precision 108-109

Type I muscles 41-42

Type II muscles 41-42

U

Ulnagrip 284

Underbar 84, **201-211**, 259,
.... 275, 282, 298-300

Underbar, Feet First 84, **201-207**, 259,
.... 275, 282, 398

Underbar, Spiral 201, **208-211**,
.... 282, 300-301

V

Values, Freerunning 31-32

Vaults 77, 84, **130-176**,
.... 259, 272, 290-295

W

Wall Dismount 177, 183, **194-196**

Wall Flip 98, **234-239**, 261,
.... 282, 300-301

Wall Run 35-36, 83, 98, 177,
.... **179-186**, 192, 259, 295, 296

Wall Spin 84, **226-233**, 259,
.... 261, 302-303

Wall Tricks 26, 84, **226-239**, 259

Wall-up 83, 179, 296

Warm-up **70-72**, 74, 262, 265, 267

WFPF 10-12, 251, 309

White skeletal muscle fibers 41

Witfeld, Jan 17, 37, 308

Woods, Shaun 242-249

World Freerunning
Parkour Federation 10-11, 251, 309

PHOTO CREDITS

Jacket photo:	Michael Schaab – www.michael-schaab.com
Jacket design:	Claudia Sakyi
Revised layout	Claudia Sakyi
Interior photos –	if not indicated otherwise:
Outdoor shots:	Michael Schaab – www.michael-schaab.com
	Ilona E. Gerling
Indoor shots:	Alexander Pach – www.move-artistic.com
Graphics:	Jonathan Haehn
	www.move-artistic.com
Graphics (pp.313-316):	Jan Witfeld, based on data collected by the German Sport University Cologne